Dr. Greg Mongeon

POWER OVER PERIMENOPAUSE

The Keys
to Treating
the Root Causes of
Your Symptoms so You
Can Get Off the Roller Coaster

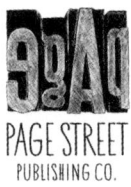

Copyright © 2026 Greg Mongeon

First published in 2026 by
Page Street Publishing Co.
27 Congress Street, Suite 1511
Salem, MA 01970
www.pagestreetpublishing.com

All rights reserved. No part of this book may be reproduced or used, in any form or by any means, electronic or mechanical, without prior permission in writing from the publisher.

Distributed by Macmillan, sales in Canada by The Canadian Manda Group.

30 29 28 27 26   1 2 3 4 5

ISBN-13: 979-8-89003-471-7

Library of Congress Control Number: 2025949491

Edited by Marissa Giambelluca
Cover and book design by Vienna Gambol for Page Street Publishing Co.

Printed and bound in China

 Page Street Publishing protects our planet by donating to nonprofits like The Trustees, which focuses on local land conservation.

Rachel, my wife of 24 years—you are the fierce love behind every risk I've taken and every dream I've dared to chase.

TABLE OF CONTENTS

Foreword   *6*

Introduction   *8*

Chapter 1

What's Going on Here? Welcome to Perimenopause   11

Chapter 2

The Journey You're Taking: Understanding Hormones   49

Chapter 3

Symptoms, Lab Tests, and the Pursuit of the Ideal Day   83

Chapter 4

Taking On Perimenopause: Build Your Protocol   112

Chapter 5

One Size Doesn't Fit All: Making Microadjustments   138

Chapter 6

Keys for Long-Term Success   162

Resources & References   *185*

Acknowledgments   *186*

About the Author   *188*

Index   *189*

Foreword

Conventional medicine introduces most women to one perspective on perimenopause. As a medical doctor who's been through perimenopause myself, I know it well. I've been on both sides of the table. The reality is that most medical doctors, even endocrinologists and ob-gyns, just aren't taught to understand hormones in a way that's comprehensive enough.

The individual hormones don't work alone—there are ratios that help us determine how they relate to one another and the lens that they should be viewed through. And beyond those hormones and their ratios, there are so many factors that ultimately impact them. Unfortunately, doctors often skim over these interactions, and many women are left with unexplained symptoms for as long as a decade—they go through perimenopause without even knowing it.

In the end, many women feel misinformed, or at least uninformed, when they leave their doctor's office. But that doesn't have to happen anymore. So much information is at our fingertips right now that just outsourcing your care to one perspective can be a bit shortsighted.

Dr. Greg isn't just giving you yet one more perspective. In this book, he walks you through a more comprehensive look at how you're living—the endocrine-disrupting chemicals in your life, the stress you experience, and the toxins you're exposed to—and then how to use this knowledge to regain power over perimenopause yourself. He lays all the cards on the table so you can understand what works best specifically for you.

Nothing about perimenopause is black and white. This entire season of life can be a gray area, and it's very nuanced. Believe me when I say I understand this time of life well, the roller coaster of symptoms. I've experienced the night sweats, the doomsday thinking, and the weight gain. I've had unexplainable headaches, and I felt myself becoming emotionally reactive. I would wake up tearful every morning. I couldn't control how I was feeling, and I couldn't explain myself to others. I felt gaslit by doctors and misunderstood by everyone else. If you're in that place, you need to know that there's hope. Today, I feel like my 20-year-old self again. I'm like a new person.

I can't overstate the importance of having this resource. You deserve to be validated and vindicated, but even more so, you deserve to be educated. If you really take the time to sit with this book, you're going to be more educated on this subject than are many doctors. You'll finally be able to advocate for yourself and start down the path to truly feeling well again.

Healing happens by taking the first step. Now is the time to get off the roller coaster and restore hope for your future. Dr. Greg is here to help.

—Jessica Peatross, MD

Introduction

Just about every day, women and men come to me with their gravest health concerns. They find me on social media by the thousands; they come into my clinic or stop me while I'm out. I've heard gut-wrenching stories from people who feel misunderstood, forgotten, or even neglected. I try to encourage them by reminding them that they are their own best advocate. I want them to know that they are empowered to start asking questions—to dig deeper and expect answers.

There's one response I get more often than not: "Dr. Greg, at this point, I don't even know which questions to ask."

Perimenopause is a natural transitory period that all women go through. Yet millions of women enter it without even knowing. Their doctor doesn't bring it up. If women broach the topic, they often hear things like "you're too young." Worse yet, the conversation's redirected: "It could be that you need to try to lose some weight."

Is this the best we have to offer for the millions of women walking into and through perimenopause? In this book, you'll learn all about the questions you need to ask. But more than that, you'll become equipped with answers. You'll reduce your reliance on outside opinions and expertise, to instead knowledgeably advocate for your own health. In time, you'll find confidence in providing your own solutions to new and lingering symptoms.

In this book, we'll also respect your individuality. We won't be so arrogant as to assume that what works for one works for all. Instead, we'll provide the key information you need to determine likely causes for what you intuitively feel and experience. With that information, we'll approach wellness protocols with proven tactics for feeling better fast. And when they don't work, we'll move into the effective troubleshooting that's often neglected.

In the not-so-distant past, I walked alongside my wife as her perimenopause journey began. In the years since, I've had thousands of conversations with women experiencing similar journeys. I've dedicated my time and attention to advanced education in the field of hormone replenishment therapy and the endocrine system. I truly want you to be well.

I'm not new to this. In two decades spent in and around health and wellness, I've had the privilege of being witness to numerous success stories. I've evaluated an almost unthinkable number of lab test panels, and I've worked on a one-on-one basis with thousands. In a conversation years ago, I was challenged to share what I knew with anyone who would listen—not just those I could see one-on-one.

Although it sounded crazy at the time, that pursuit led me to posting walk-and-talk videos on TikTok. Through social media, I now have the privilege of speaking to tens of millions who view my videos. Better yet, I hear their stories. They share their pain with me, and I have the opportunity to empathize with them. But there's something else—in time, the success stories started coming, from women and men who applied a principle from a one-minute video on their social media feed and transformed their lives.

The women I hear from most often are those who find themselves in the midst of perimenopause or menopause. I hope my videos help them kick in the right direction, but I wrote this book to be more than a kickoff. My aim is for this guide to bring you from day one all the way through into a successful transition to menopause.

This is not a setup. There isn't a "gotcha" moment, or a secret sauce behind closed doors. I firmly believe that if you read and apply these time-tested principles, you will make significant strides toward feeling like the real you again. I say it with confidence because I've seen it happen. The women and their loved ones who have come to me with heartfelt thanks for the transformation they've experienced are my motivation to share what I know to be true with you in this book. I'm looking forward to taking this journey together.

Dr. Greg

1.
WHAT'S GOING ON HERE? WELCOME TO PERIMENOPAUSE

Did you know there are languages that don't have specific words to encapsulate what we know as "menopause" or "perimenopause?" In certain cultures, this phase of life is celebrated as a gentle transition. In others, westernization only just now demands the creation of new words to capture what it means to have such a symptom as a "hot flash."

Even in the Western world, it's estimated that 20 percent of women walk through perimenopause completely symptom-free. [1] Wow. Does that sound like you?

If you've been led to believe that perimenopause is a standard, uniform experience for all women of a certain age, let me be the first to apologize on behalf of the health community. If this were the case, as we're often led to believe, why would every woman experience it so differently? Couldn't the pain, symptoms, and frustration be alleviated with a quick run to the hormone clinic?

Misconceptions, Lies, and Culture on Perimenopause

Seventy-five million Americans woke up this morning in the thick of perimenopause. That's roughly 20 percent of the entire country's population. So, why do you feel alone? Why do doctors seem largely unable to meaningfully guide women through this time of life, while minimizing the symptoms they experience?

Information is hard to come by, and a lot of the resources you do find contradict one another. One doctor tells you to consider hormone replacement therapy, the next tells you it will give you cancer. And I'll bet your doctor isn't the only voice in your head. Your friends have opinions, social media creators have opinions, everyone has an opinion!

And yet, you may still feel alone. Why is that? Part of it is shame: You may be experiencing symptoms that are out of your comfort zone for discussion with others. And if you never bring them up, you never come to understand that other women are walking through similar experiences right alongside you.

Worse yet, maybe you *have* brought up your concerns, and a doctor or friend has left you feeling dismissed and confused. There are a few go-to responses women in perimenopause get. See whether you can check off all four:

- Your lab test results are normal.
- This just comes with aging.
- Consider losing weight.
- There's nothing I can do for you.

Any of these hit a little too close to home? You're tired of it, I'm tired of it . . . so let's forge a different way forward.

The Journey We're Taking

If we were taking a hike together, you'd probably want to know a few things before you agreed to set out: Where are we going? How arduous is the trail? How long?

I can only imagine some of the same emotions arise as you read the first pages of this book. While your friends and traditional doctors may just shrug off perimenopause, these are the days of TikTok and Instagram, so you're probably acquainted with armchair experts as well.

This book does not offer an "Easy" button. I reject the notion that there's one hidden tool, tactic, capsule, pill, or nutrient I could reveal to you that would instantly override your symptoms and restore your quality of life. But, that said, I do believe we can do it together. I ask your willingness to learn the *why*, so that I can teach you the *how*.

Here's the core belief that informs this book: I simply can't accept that this natural, beautiful transition that all women will walk through requires debilitating symptoms. But at the same time, I acknowledge that these symptoms are very real.

Every woman's body is different, but success leaves clues. And when our clients step out at the end of the journey that my team and I lead them through, they report success. They report reduced or eliminated symptoms, healthier mindsets, and better results in lab testing.

So, if perimenopause is natural, why do the symptoms seem unnatural?

You've Been Through This Before . . . Kind Of

When a little girl is born, there are virtually no hormones in her body. And then, all of a sudden, as early as at the age of 9 or 10, she gets hit with something called puberty. And what happens at that point is that hormones go on a crazy roller coaster ride. If you're a parent reading this, you're probably thinking that you're well aware and could write the book on that.

Interestingly enough, perimenopause mirrors this experience in some ways. A woman straps back in for round two of the hormone roller coaster. The reason that it's a bigger deal this time is due to something called *life accumulation*. Life accumulation is exactly what it sounds like—all of the life you've lived stacking up against you to make the fight harder. Think of it as a bucket capturing rainwater while it slowly fills to the brim.

Once puberty ends, you march into the rest of your teenage years. All in all, this is a hormonally stable time of life, compared to puberty. But even then, you're capturing rainwater. You're exposed to viruses and toxins, establishing a diet, and perhaps even using products like makeup or other body care. The point isn't to lament every unwise decision, but to consider how an empty bucket begins to fill for each of us.

The same teenage effect rolls into your 20s, your 30s, and then, of course, you get to present day looking at a much different scenario than the one you experienced during the hormonal swings in your early years.

Think about all the stress that your body has been through in all this time. The body has a bad tendency of holding on to stress of all forms—chemical, physical, emotional, mental, environmental, and so on. When the hormone roller coaster meets that stored stress? Fireworks.

By the way, many women experience a similar effect during or after pregnancy. Anecdotally, it seems that a lot of them notice a greater effect after the birth of their second or third child, even if the first pregnancy and postpartum period went smoothly. Just like the hormonal shifts caused by perimenopause, the hormonal shifts resulting from pregnancy can stir up all kinds of craziness as the body responds.

But I truly believe it doesn't have to be this way. I believe we can address the overflowing bucket and restore the sheriff in town. We can experience the hormonal fluctuations without the symptoms associated with them.

The Cause of Symptoms During Perimenopause

Years ago, I started noticing a pattern emerging. I've evaluated thousands upon thousands of lab testing results. I've hosted consultations and appointments with numerous perimenopausal women. Here's what I believe: When a woman enters perimenopause, the drastic shift stirs up things that previously lay dormant in the body. These chronic conditions, autoimmune diseases, and other issues yet to be realized come to the surface just as the endocrine system shifts. You can only imagine the consequences—or maybe you're experiencing them right now!

Studies are confirming my convictions. In 2019, the peer-reviewed journal *Frontiers in Endocrinology* published a piece authored by Maunil K. Desai and Roberta Diaz Brinton. Check out what they say in its abstract: "[E]ndocrine transitions exert profound impact on the development of autoimmune diseases in women through complex mechanisms. Greater understanding of endocrine transitions and their role in autoimmune diseases could aid in prediction, prevention, and cures of these debilitating diseases in women." [2]

And here's the thing: It doesn't stop with autoimmune disease! A growing body of research suggests that perimenopause carries with it massive neurological ramifications. It can impact bone health, heart health, gut health, and more.

But enough with the doom and gloom. I actually love knowing the root cause of symptoms. Once we know the root cause, we can treat *that* instead of racing to patch up bullet wounds with Band-Aids®. We're not looking for a silver bullet, though. There's not a single diagnosis to pursue or a bottle of supplements that will make all your problems go away. But if we find the causes and treat them (yes, *them*, as in more than one), we can win the battle, reduce your symptoms, and restore your quality of life.

How'd We Get Here?

Picture again an image I brought up earlier—a rain barrel filled to the brim. This is the life accumulation we discussed. It's all of the stress your body has been carrying unawares through the years. Suddenly, someone brings over a bucket of something called perimenopause, and dumps it out into that full rain barrel. Now, we're dealing with overflow, and you're definitely aware of it.

Symptoms spring up, lab test markers go haywire, and you are now on a hormonal roller coaster. Some women truly feel as if their life has fallen apart. Maybe you relate—your skin changes, your hair's falling out, and every muscle aches. You feel as if you've lost a step as your brain becomes foggy and you find it difficult to concentrate. Maybe you're dealing with poor sleep, urinary tract infections (UTIs), mood swings, or low libido. We haven't even touched the many changes you're experiencing within your menstrual cycle.

If this describes you, my heart goes out to you. You need to know that there's hope. The women who come into my clinic feeling the way you feel do see transformation. They do see symptoms minimize or disappear. Perimenopause will always bring fluctuating hormones, but there don't have to be symptoms and chaos along the way.

Take a moment to reflect on the life that you've lived that brought you to this point. Have you birthed children? Battled illness? Dealt with intense emotional stress from jobs, relationships, or family? Have you been exposed to toxins or consumed them in your food? *By the way, the answer to that one is almost certainly yes.*

I could go on and on. Take an inventory of the stress you've experienced in your life. This could be anything, like moving around a lot as a kid or later in life, bearing financial burdens, experiencing disordered eating, or losing a loved one.

Those stresses are nothing to be ashamed of. We've all had our rain barrels filled up to some extent over the course of our lives. My wife and I have five kids—she spent large portions of a decade and a half either pregnant or nursing. That's a blessing, but it's also a lot to ask of a woman's body.

Have grace for yourself. The point in taking a stress inventory isn't to get down on life, it's simply to understand where you are now. Everything you can identify helps point to the source of your symptoms and gives us clues about what we can address together. There are people who would see more benefit from unpacking past emotional pain than from taking any supplement!

There's a physical, mental, emotional, and spiritual part of any healing journey. And this isn't woo-woo. I'm not going to ask you to do anything that will have you raising an eyebrow. This is a line of thinking confirmed in studies that have been performed and embraced by the medical community at large. If you're having doubts, look into the incredible research surrounding adverse childhood events, as just one reference point. The Cleveland Clinic offers a research-backed overview of the topic in an impactful resource that's well worth reviewing. It's cited along with the other references in this book. [3]

Medicine vs This Book

I have dedicated over twenty years to learning the field of functional medicine. In my opinion, this health-care philosophy is the sweet spot between conventional Western medicine and traditional holistic health principles. My functional medicine background informs the way I approach perimenopause with the thousands of women who have come through the doors of my clinic in this stage of life.

Similarities

Let's start with the ways my approach is similar to the Western medicine approach, and then we'll talk about the differences. The part of my process that will be familiar to most anyone who's stepped foot in a doctor's office is lab testing. I truly believe that, in this day and age, medical-grade lab testing is essential for understanding our starting point. If we can pinpoint where you stand today with accurate, reliable data, we can understand how it is that your body is feeling the impact.

Medical-grade lab tests reveal not just an explanation for symptoms, but also provide insight into root causes. We can't look at each marker individually and try to resolve high or low levels for each. We must look at the test results as being a bird's-eye view of you, and that means considering how each one of these elements that appear to be independent markers on a sheet of paper are actually key to how your body functions. Every one interacts somewhere in your body, creating an intricate, complex system.

Key Differences

Believe it or not, we've already reached the end of the similarities to the conventional medicine approach. Respectfully, I thank God for conventional Western medicine. I'd be a widower without it. I witnessed my wife pulled into an emergency C-section that saved not only her life, but that of my newborn as well. Western medicine plays an essential role, and I'm grateful for it.

You could probably assume this, but the United States is the best place in the world to be if you ever have need of emergency medical services. If I'm in a car accident, please don't call a functional medicine doctor. Call the ambulance, save my life! Unfortunately, we have another reputation as a country—we're ranked among the lowest in terms of how we handle long-standing, chronic conditions and symptoms.

So, when we look at perimenopause, we need to understand and appreciate that, to see results, we can't keep going with the status quo. What got us here won't get us there. That leads me back into how the approach to perimenopause outlined in this book will differ from conventional medicine.

I say this as respectfully as possible, but medical doctors graduate and come into the field with a specific toolkit. To oversimplify, that toolkit is essentially prescriptions and surgeries. Think about it—if you go to your doctor with a concern and don't come back with a "something" to take that will solve your symptoms, are you satisfied with the visit?

If you have a doctor who takes the time to provide lifestyle recommendations and give advice, I give them massive credit for doing so within the boundaries of a broken system that demands shorter and shorter patient interactions. Because here's the elephant in the room—research published in *Health Services Research* suggests the average primary-care physician is likely spending no more than 10 minutes in the room with you, having no more than 5 minutes to dedicate to your reason for your visit. [4] Wow.

What if we took the same lab tests utilized in the medical system, but came to them with a different approach? What if we weren't limited by expectations for a doctor's appointment or an approach that seeks only to patch symptoms as they arise? I invite you to consider embracing the root-cause approach.

My favorite part of what I do is being curious. In my initial consultation, I will spend 45 minutes digging deep. We start from birth (if possible) and cover the major milestones in your life. We dig deep into the symptoms you're experiencing, seeking patterns and correlations. Then, we order the right lab tests and consider them from a wildly different perspective than may your regular doctor.

Armed with reliable data and an optimal-health mindset, we seek to understand the causes behind the symptoms. We leave nothing off the table in our approach. Some of the tools we use are God's and your grandma's—those lifestyle tweaks that cost you nothing but commitment. You'll learn how to breathe correctly to reset your nervous system. We'll incorporate manageable movement and make the essential tweaks to your nutrition plan. We'll explore powerful, researched modalities and such tools as red light therapy, infrared, lymphatic massage, castor oil packs, and many more. We'll look at supplements and hormone replacement therapy as well—and we'll do it in a way that's completely different from anything you've heard before.

The foundational protocol we craft together in this book will first help you restore natural energy and revitalize your drainage system. It will help optimize and balance your hormones, and it will provide much-needed support to your immune system. We'll talk about how such organs as your gut, thyroid, liver, kidneys, and others come to the table, and what to do if lab results suggest any are stressed or struggling.

Sound like a plan? Let's dig in.

Perimenopause vs Menopause

First things first: Let's agree on some definitions. Although it might sound simple, keep in mind that many doctors fail to define when a woman has entered perimenopause. There's a false belief that this time of life is mostly defined by being of a certain age, but in reality, perimenopause can affect women in a wide age spectrum ranging from the mid-30s to the mid-50s. You might go well into your 40s before you begin perimenopause, but it could hit others as much as a decade sooner.

So, if it's not identifiable by age, how is it defined? Perimenopause is a time when menstrual cycles become irregular. Unlike menopause, perimenopause can last as long as a decade. It's characterized by the beginning of symptoms we typically associate with menopause. Apart from your periods becoming irregular, you may notice symptoms ranging from insomnia to joint pain, vaginal dryness, low libido, or even mood swings. The list of potential symptoms goes on and on. As we addressed back on page 12, some women go through perimenopause symptom-free, whereas others may experience completely debilitating symptoms.

The symptoms are caused by hormone fluctuations as a transitory period begins.

If that's perimenopause, what is menopause itself? Menopause is more clearly defined—you have entered it at the point when you have gone a full 12 months without having a menstrual cycle. Perimenopause is the precursor to menopause.

Don't Skip the Foundation

I've been around the block a few times, and I've seen numerous women make the attempt to skip to the place in our process that seems to offer the biggest payoff. I've seen the desperate search for the "Easy" button . . . or at least the "Instant" button.

The problem is, that's not the way our body works. Believe it or not, our body is designed to heal. That's the dose of hope I have for you as you dig through these early pages. Here's the rest of the statement: Our body is designed to heal; *it just needs no interference.* I believe with every fiber of my being that everything we do together isn't about attempting to heal ourselves—it's about removing the interference and kick-starting our body's natural healing process.

Allowing our body to heal itself gives us an advantage—we can avoid the painful process of constantly tweaking and tinkering with a protocol that keeps everything at bay. Instead, we just trust our body. But that's not to say we won't come alongside our body to do some critical work that allows that process to start firing on all cylinders.

Resist TikTok, Instagram, and Your Friends

I appreciate the irony here. If you've ever joined me for a "walk and talk" on TikTok or Instagram, you know that I love speaking to people on social media. I have a "give away the farm" mentality, and I don't hold back on the value I'm willing to share. I'm grateful for the many other health experts who do the same.

But here's where we need to be mindful—social media content can be convincing and compelling. Sometimes, these videos (or our friends who've seen them) convince us that the missing key has been found. They get us to overhaul our pantry or stuff our supplement cabinet and throw all our eggs into the proverbial basket.

What I need to tell you is that it's possible to do the right thing at the wrong time. I also need you to know that if a silver bullet existed, we'd all be aware of it.

Yet how many impulse buys have you made on TikTok? How many podcast clips have you saved on Instagram? These fancy, elaborate gimmicks all seem to promise instant healing.

Can you really skip out on the fundamentals, start avoiding lectins, and see your health completely transform? Come on, let's be real!

I'd love to offer just one suggestion: Stay the course. Don't be diverted into thinking that you can toss out your comprehensive protocol in exchange for an influencer's hack. You can pencil down their ideas to experiment with at a later date, but none of it's going to make any difference for you until you've laid the foundation.

Take a State of the Union

We've finally arrived. We're ready to start this journey together. Before we do, I urge you to take what I like to call a State of the Union. This exercise is a head-to-toe self-analysis. What I want you to do is be observant and mindful. Consider each individual element of your body more deeply than you typically do, and write down a detailed observation of what you find.

Here's how to do it: Start from the top of your head and work your way down to your toes. On the top of your head, you find your hair and scalp. How's your hair doing? Is it as soft and luscious as it's always been, or has it turned dry and brittle? Is it falling out in clumps or excessively oily? Is your scalp dry and itchy? Consider every possible detail you can, and then work your way inside to your brain.

Are you thinking clearly or plagued with brain fog? Do you find yourself searching for words or forgetting names you should know? Is stress impacting your thoughts? How's your self-talk?

Keep working your way down your body, and don't skip anything. Capture the state of your skin, nails, joints . . . everything!

Why is this important? For multiple reasons. The first is that some of us don't even realize our State of the Union until we take the time to thoroughly assess it. In doing this, some of us may notice symptoms we're experiencing that we hadn't even fully realized.

By the way, your State of the Union should capture more than just symptoms. Ideally, you'll also capture the major life circumstances that could be impacting your health in unexpected ways. If you're married or have kids, how are those relationships? Do you feel supported or abandoned? How's work? Is your daily routine draining you?

It might seem silly to track things that aren't directly tied to physical health, but countless studies show the relationship between stress in any form and physical symptoms. Don't leave anything off the table; everything can be a clue and everything's worth tracking.

Compiling and keeping a State of the Union is also essential because, as things begin to improve, many people fail to even remember where they came from. Different steps along the way can feel frustrating, and we start telling ourselves lies that we feel no better than we did when we started. A thorough pre-analysis helps with this.

Later on, we're going to walk through an "Ideal Day" exercise together. When we do, your State of the Union exercise will be helpful to inform it.

Prime Your Nervous System for Healing

The nervous system doesn't spend a lot of time in the limelight. But lately, one important piece of it has been popularized. You may have heard someone talk about being stuck in a "fight-or-flight" state. That's not just a mindset; that's actually a state the nervous system can be in, called the *sympathetic* state. In this state, the body actually launches into a physiological response appropriate for self-defense or preservation.

The Fight-or-Flight Nervous System

This natural response can actually be amazingly beneficial. If you were being chased by a bear, you'd want your nervous system to launch into the sympathetic state. What's happening is that all of your body's focus is rechanneled toward only the essential functions that help you survive. It gives you more "juice" in some key areas, by eliminating or reducing its work in other areas. Here's the not-so-amazing part—your body can't distinguish one form of stress from another. It can't tell the difference between being chased by a bear and dealing with everyday stress at home. If you're experiencing stress of any form, it's likely that you're launched into the sympathetic state.

You may be caught in this state chronically. And here's the problem: This is not a healing state. This is a survival state. There are implications for your digestion, your heart, your liver, your eyes, and your lungs. [5] Let's put it this way: There's not a nutrient or hormone on earth you could be given in this state that would work as effectively as it should, unless you can come out of this chronically sympathetic condition.

We'll provide some tools, but before we do, let's understand the two other states of the nervous system, so you can identify another place where you may be and then, ultimately, where you hope to go.

The Frozen Nervous System

We just looked at the term "fight or flight." You may be familiar with the full phrase, which is actually "fight, flight, or freeze." Despite what I was taught in my doctoral program years ago, there actually is a state of the nervous system that encompasses the "freeze" portion of that statement. The *dorsal vagal* state of the nervous system, sometimes called the dorsal vagal shutdown, is kicked into gear when the body is under an extreme state of stress. For instance, if you genuinely believe your life is at risk, you may fall into this shutdown state. Your body is saying, "Stick a fork in me, I'm done."

As the sympathetic state's efforts are effectively shut down, you prepare to accept your fate. Symptoms may actually decrease during this time as the body becomes less sensitive to them. Here's the problem—other symptoms pick up steam. Symptoms like depression, fatigue, and brain fog. This is not a state we want our body to be in.

The final state of the nervous system is where we're setting our sights. The *parasympathetic* state is the place where your body needs to be for you to "rest, digest, and heal." It sounds like a beautiful reality, because it is. We have tools and tactics that can help you return to this state, but for now, I'm going to leave you with just one. It's my favorite combination of effective and completely free.

Changing Your State with Breathwork

The way you breathe matters, and you're probably doing it wrong. This incredible, simple process we all take for granted has the ability to make a major impact on the body. The fastest way I know of to reset the state of your nervous system is by utilizing breathwork.

The topic of breathwork is surprisingly well researched and offers many benefits. There are numerous different techniques and tactics, but I'm going to teach you the simplest of them. The tactic we're going to learn today is box breathing. Picture a square—each side of the square represents four seconds. The first thing we're going to do is take a deep nasal breath—you're going to breathe in for a full four seconds. Then, hold that breath in for four seconds. Follow that up by exhaling for a full four seconds, and holding the breath out for a full four seconds.

That's one box. Your goal is to string 20 boxes together. If this feels painfully slow and time-consuming . . . you probably need it. That moment of slowing down, breathing correctly, and chilling out is what your nervous system needs. You can try doing this every night before bed or every morning after waking. But the reality is you can do it anytime—maybe on the drive to or from work, or in the shower.

Breathing is like drinking water. It sounds too simple, so many people become disinterested. I urge you not to skip this step. Find a place to incorporate breathwork into your routine. Stick with it long enough and see whether you experience a difference.

The Journey Starts Now: Time to Ditch the Symptoms

Let's be honest, you've been reading about laying a foundation. Now we're here, and you're bracing yourself for me to throw you under the bus for your diet and lifestyle. That's not what we're doing. I'll be honest: You may need to make some lifestyle tweaks, but that's not what this section is about.

Most women have already been thrown under the bus for diet and lifestyle. And here's the thing—some of them didn't deserve it! You wouldn't believe how many times I've had patients tell me, "Dr. Greg, here's my diet. Here's my workout plan. Here's me. Explain." Despite what you've been told, there are more layers in wellness than just nutrition.

So, where do we begin? With these two key elements:

- Producing clean, natural, sustainable energy
- Promoting efficient, effective drainage

That's it! If it sounds elementary, you need to hear this: Most women find that addressing nothing more or less than these two things completely changes their quality of life. These are cornerstones in your journey. You can't make it through the rest without them. Virtually no healing protocol will be effective if even one of the two is lagging behind.

Stick with me through the rest of this chapter, and I'll leave you with a way to get some early wins under your belt so you can start feeling better fast.

Aren't We Forgetting Something?

Hold on—you may be thinking, "We're diving in to create an action plan, but nothing about producing energy and promoting drainage sounds like a hormone conversation." I didn't forget about hormones, and there's a very specific reason that we start here.

In the next couple of chapters of this book, I'll introduce you to tools that can have a mind-blowing effect toward your goal of hormone balance, replenishment, and optimization. I've been studying in this area for years, and I've recently become certified in advanced bioidentical hormone replacement therapy in a postdoctoral program. Trust me when I say we're not afraid to talk hormones.

But what I need you to know is that you can't plant a rose in a garden bed filled with weeds. If we're going to grow a flourishing garden, we have to do more than just plant the seeds; we have to prime the soil. The body responds appropriately to its environment. So, if the body is responding to something, what's in the environment?

At a glance, you might just assume that your body has gone haywire. But in over 20 years practicing functional medicine, I've learned to appreciate the intelligence of the body, and I personally don't believe it goes haywire nearly as often as conventional medicine would have us assume. What if there are factors at play invisible to the human eye, yet 100 percent real?

Is your end goal for your hormones to show the appropriate numbers in a follow-up visit with your doctor, or is it to feel well, act well, think well, and be well? If your goal is to truly become well, we need to look at your body as one cohesive unit, rather than as thousands of individual pieces.

Why This Starting Point?

If you want to drive a car, you better be sure you have gas in the tank. The same is true for your body! If you want to tackle the challenges brought up by hormonal shifts and all that got stirred up along with that shift, you need cellular energy. Cellular energy, also known as ATP, fuels essentially every bodily process. If you're walking around feeling depleted and exhausted after a full night's sleep, you very likely lack sufficient cellular energy for optimal function.

Go back to grade school science with me for a moment. We all learned that our mitochondria are the powerhouse of our cells. What they don't teach you is that this statement was recently discovered to be only a partial truth.

Dr. Robert Naviaux introduced us to a theory called the cell danger response (CDR). To oversimplify his incredible body of research, a key finding was that mitochondria are indeed the powerhouse of our cells . . . sometimes. In other cases, when our body encounters a threat of some nature, the mitochondria launch into an incredible sequence of processes that essentially turn us into a battleship. Our cells are quite literally prepared for war, and attention is diverted from energy production into this defense mechanism. [6]

So, what does that mean? It means that if your body is under attack from chronic infection, chronic toxicity, or something similar, it can't produce energy as effectively. This complicates the cellular energy conversation, because we have to respect this reality. It's a sobering revelation that we can't simply supply nutrients; we must also consider whether we need to simultaneously support our body in handling the invasion.

No wonder you're exhausted! Since everything else collapses without sufficient cellular energy, this is the very first step we take with every client at our clinic . . . regardless of diagnosis. The same is true for perimenopause, when we find that women come to us depleted of energy.

Here's the good news: This foundational step in the journey has many women feeling better, stronger, and more energetic in a remarkably short period of time.

Producing Clean, Natural Energy . . . Quickly!

Let's get your energy levels back up, so you can feel like you again. What I love about addressing energy levels is that there's a compound effect. Not only do you physically feel better, but your cells, themselves, are actually bolstered with energy. If your cells are starved of nutrients, they can't produce energy. If they can't produce energy, you certainly won't succeed in offsetting that with more energy drinks and coffee.

Cellular energy (ATP) is sensitive to a number of inputs. Some of them are the typical standbys in the health and wellness world; others may be new to you.

You Only *Think* You're Hydrated

I know you're tempted to skip this section. Most people try to skip the topic even when they're directly asked about it. In an initial consultation, most people will flag themselves as well hydrated. It's not until I make them quantify what that means that we can come to the mutual understanding that their body is severely dehydrated.

Trust me when I say that if the majority of the American population were well hydrated, I'd gladly skip this section and get to the more interesting parts. But I urge you to actually track your water intake for a day, in comparison to how much water you should be drinking. If, at that point, you can stand behind your water intake with confidence, you earn the green checkmark here. But my guess would be that about 80 percent of people only think they're hydrated. You may give yourself a pass here because you've *heard* this information before, not because you live it.

Drinking enough water isn't easy at first. It's okay to increase day by day until you've reached the target. You might find that bathroom habits change or that you feel almost "waterlogged" at first, but in time your body will adjust and normalize. Most people will ultimately feel much better once they've adjusted to the changes.

Revamping Your Diet the Almost Painless Way

There are two easy ways to get nutrients into your body on a daily basis. One way to absorb nutrients is via the food that you eat. The other way to get nutrients is via supplementation. If you have other options available to you, such as IV therapy, you're welcome to explore those as well! But in this section, we'll focus on diet and supplements.

An article by Matthew Solan in the *Harvard Health Blog* summarizes the dietary needs for ATP production concisely: "Boost your ATP with fatty acids and protein . . . ." [7] Sounds easy enough, right? Like drinking more water, it's harder than it sounds at times! But once you get the routine going, it gets easier.

This is not just a diet and exercise book. You could wear a blindfold and still find plenty of those at your local bookstore or library. I want to make another distinction in tandem with that one: This is not a crazy sauce supplement cabinet world, either. Most people need to slim down their supplement cabinet, not beef it up.

But both dietary modifications and supplements have their place within the broader category of lifestyle modification. We can't ignore them, and in fact, we can gain massive benefits from them. Neither is the "Easy" button, nor is either the silver bullet—but you can make leaps and bounds by having both in your toolkit.

Let's start with your diet. Many, many people have told you all about what not to eat. Right now, I want to focus on what *to* eat. What you may find is that the more you incorporate those elements, the less room you have in your diet for the things your body isn't benefiting from.

Protein intake is essential and, in my opinion, it's the number one thing women lack in their typical diet. The protein you consume should come from good-quality sources. I am not afraid of grass-fed, grass-finished red meat!

There's no way around this—meat is probably the best and most easily available source of protein. If you can, incorporate more of it into your diet. Other good sources of protein include Greek yogurt, pasture-raised eggs, high-quality cheese, and fish.

By the way, after protein, fatty acids are one of the most important nutrients to get to your cells for the purpose of energy production. The great thing is that many of the foods containing fatty acids go well with the protein foods from the first list, or even overlap. Find a grass-fed butter or tallow. Otherwise, turn to coconut oil and olive oil. Nuts, seeds, and fish are all excellent sources for fatty acids.

Notice that, here, we're talking about wellness by addition. I haven't asked you to remove even one thing from your diet. What you'll find is that the closer you get to an ideal protein intake, the more the worst parts of your diet will be crowded out naturally. You may have to specifically sacrifice certain guilty pleasures if you're out of balance with them, but addition is the best place to start.

Are you ready for your target? It's a big one—aim for 1 gram of protein consumed per pound of body weight. So, if you weigh 170 pounds (77 kg), you're trying to get in 170 grams of protein. Some quick math might show you that you're a long way from that! On the bright side, that might explain some of that fatigue you've been experiencing.

Your Supplements Aren't Doing You Any Favors … But They Should Be

Supplements describe themselves accurately. The purpose of a supplement is to complement an already healthy diet—not replace one. Try as you might, you can't out-supplement a crappy diet. Many have tried before you.

As much as I appreciate seeing people begin to understand and appreciate the role of a good-quality supplement, you need to know that your jam-packed supplement cabinet isn't doing you any favors. Most of those supplements should be thrown out. Some are bad quality; others are good for you and *still* need to be thrown out. Why? Because there can be too much of a good thing.

What I've found is that excessive supplementation can actually become a stressor to the body. Whatever benefit the nutrients inside offer is counteracted by the sheer stress the body goes through by needing to digest and deal with them all. You also need to know that supplements can take time to make a difference! Cycling onto one thing and off another every time the bottle empties out is counterproductive unless you're being mindful of a larger strategy.

So, when it comes to cellular energy, what nutrients are required from supplements to move the needle? Let's take another look at our body's cells. We know that cellular energy is produced by our mitochondria. By eating sufficient protein and fatty acids, we're providing fuel to that process. But we can go a layer deeper.

While protein and fatty acid intake supplies the primary source of fuel for our cells, we can make their process of creating energy more efficient. If I were buying a supplement to support my mitochondria, I'd look for antioxidants on the ingredient label. We'll keep this light, so you aren't tempted to reach for your bookmark, but it helps to understand free radicals at a basic level. Free radicals are unstable molecules that can be found in all bodies. If they aren't neutralized, they damage cells, decrease organ function, and even impact our DNA.

This is the major reason you hear so much about antioxidants. Antioxidants are known to neutralize these free radicals, preventing all of that damage from occurring. You can see how neutralizing free radicals can aid in the cellular energy production process!

Supplement science is moving quickly, but as of the writing of this book, some of the top antioxidants for cellular energy are n-acetyl cysteine (NAC), alpha lipoic acid (ALA), acetyl-L-carnitine (ALC), and resveratrol. A good mitochondrial support supplement will have one or more of these ingredients, plus quality cellular micronutrients that feed the energy production process.

In the supplement world, it's worth doing the research to ensure you can trust the brand that you're buying a product from. Many brands will add a microdose of a buzzword ingredient so that they can claim it on the label. You don't need to be a scientist or deeply researched on supplements to make more informed decisions. Run a couple of quick online searches for the key ingredients. Simply search "effective dose of [ingredient name]," so you can get an idea of what you're looking for.

By the way, I want to help you navigate the crazy Wild West of the supplement world. I mentioned earlier that supplement science is moving so quickly that I can't even put my best recommendations to paper inside this book; instead, the Resources section (page 185) includes a URL that will take you to my recommendations. Please note that I am not a pitch man for any one supplement company—I actually utilize a variety of brands, because my goal is to get the best of the best, regardless of the name on the label.

Stop Overcomplicating Exercise

First, we talked about water intake; then, we talked about your diet; and now, we're talking about exercise? What could be worse! Before you jump to conclusions, I want you to know that I see you. If you have no desire to work out, you're not lazy. Maybe you need to read that again to believe it—you're not lazy. Your body is fighting a battle, and your energy is depleted. Of course, you don't feel like hitting the gym.

You may do it anyway, and if so, I applaud you for that. Or you may be physically unable . . . and that's okay, too. There's a term I use inside my clinic: "manageable movement." Emphasis on *manageable*. The great thing about manageable movement is it's not a workout protocol. I'm not going to provide a list of daily exercises complete with the reps to do for each.

Manageable movement is different for all of us. You have one mission, and it's quite simply to move your body. Don't live within your comfort zone, but don't push yourself too far, either. Find the healthy balance. If you're accustomed to spending evenings on the couch, try a walk around the block. Don't lay any added pressure on yourself to cover a certain distance or achieve a particular heart rate.

You just need to move. Move more than you're used to moving, but don't burn yourself out. Don't compare yourself to your friends, and scroll on past when you see a fitness influencer on social media. As cellular energy is restored, your capacity will come back with it. But it's a chicken-and-the-egg scenario—movement requires cellular energy, but it also helps in the production of it.

By the way, gym rats, a quick word for you as well. I'm a fan of working out and I'm a fan of the gym. But I need you to know that chronic cardio can have a negative impact on your body. It's absolutely possible that you're overdoing it and causing stress that contributes to the symptoms you experience. Incorporate rest into your weekly gym routine to see greater benefits and better balance.

The Secret to Sleeping Well

This alone could be the topic for another book. This likely won't be the last time we address sleep, but we'll dive in with a brief introduction. We've all heard that sleep matters, but most of us continue to show a complete lack of respect for just how impactful it is. Quality sleep is literally essential for survival.

And here's the problem—that's easy to say. You may already be yelling at me right now. Because as much as experts love to tell you how important sleep is, they seem to be short on how to optimize it.

Before we dive in to a few sleep-related tips and tricks, I want to acknowledge that major hormonal components are at play in many cases of insomnia. And the problems extend past just the hormonal; sometimes, organ stress even causes an inability to sleep restfully.

Later on, we're going to dig into that and help you identify whether these factors contribute to your insomnia journey. But for now, let's cover some sleep recommendations that can benefit everyone. I probably don't even need to say it, but replenishing sleep is quite obviously a major key for producing cellular energy. So, how do you set the stage for restorative sleep?

Here's a cheat sheet:
- Eat your last bite of food 3 hours before sleeping.
- No screens 2 hours before bed.
- Get your bedroom pitch black.
- Get your bedroom cold—under 68°F (20°C), if possible.
- Create a winding-down routine and/or try journaling.
- Try mouth taping.

I get it; that's a laundry list. You don't have to implement all of this at once, but try a few tips that resonate with you. As we go through several things here, you'll find that your nervous system and brain are primary points of interest in the sleep conversation. There's actually some good science here. For instance, the reason you want to eat your last bite of food a few hours before bedtime is so that food isn't being digested in the middle of the night. Your glymphatic system, which essentially drains your brain of toxins, works best at night. And if your body has to digest food at night, attention is diverted from the essential task of sleeping.

We also know that flickering blue light from screens stimulates your pineal gland. The pineal gland tells your body that it's time to be awake! Sounds counterproductive, right?

It's also for the sake of your brain and nervous system that I advocate for a pitch-black room or a sleep mask. Believe it or not, even a pinprick of light from a smoke detector or light peeking in from behind the curtains creates information for your brain to process. A very interesting neurological conversation occurs there.

A cold bedroom is another important element. Although it may sound like nothing more than a preference, a cold bedroom actually promotes sleep. When you're trying to fall asleep, your body temperature actually drops—and a cold bedroom supports this process.

Why do I recommend a winding-down routine or journaling? So many women report that the number one reason they can't sleep is anxiety or a mind that's racing. Journaling is a good way to soothe the mind. You could even try a gratitude journal and focus on only the things that you're most grateful for. If you're a person of prayer, it's a great time to pray. Right before bed is an excellent time to practice breathwork (page 28) as well.

As for mouth taping—is that what it sounds like? You bet it is. Using micropore tape or other tapes designed specifically for this task, you simply cover your mouth and assist your body in prioritizing nasal breathing at night. This can be very impactful, and many people report a better quality of sleep as a result. You get used to it faster than you think, and eventually you might not want to go without it!

We're Not Done with Energy

We finished the cellular energy crash course, but we're not done with the topic. This is so integral to your success on a perimenopause healing journey that I don't want to just pass over it quickly. We'll dive in with more tools and tactics later on, so stay tuned. And above all, don't kick these fundamentals to the curb in favor of "fancier" things that sound new and novel. The advanced therapies won't work without the foundation.

In Chapter 4 (page 112), we'll help you build a comprehensive protocol with this in mind. But in the meantime, feel free to start with what we've already covered.

Drainage: Opening Up the Body's Exit Doors

Cellular energy is just one of my two foundational steps that everything else is built on top of. The second step in the conversation is drainage. "Drainage" refers to the way things leave the body. If you've ever heard terminology surrounding detoxes and cleanses, drainage is what those protocols seek to promote.

Think of drainage as involving a funnel: Things come into the body, and your body intelligently removes what it doesn't find useful. The problem with a funnel is that a clog at any point inside it will cause a backup. Next thing you know, the nasty, useless things your body is carrying can't escape. And then? Overflow. This overflow could consist of anything from undigested food particles to heavy metals, toxins, fluids, bile, and more.

Seven pieces work together to form this drainage funnel, and if even one is functioning suboptimally, the whole thing can overflow. The pieces of the drainage funnel are:

- Gut
- Liver
- Kidneys
- Lymphatic system
- Glymphatic system
- Sweat glands
- Respiratory system

Each of these individual systems is responsible for filtering different things out of the body. Sometimes, processes overlap. For instance, there's no hole in your right rib cage underneath your liver! The liver relies on the gut to complete the job of draining toxins and more out of the body.

If the whole drainage funnel is working as it should, you'll feel better. Absolutely no doubt about it. As a bonus, you clear the way for other health protocols to become much more effective.

Identifying Sluggish Drainage

There could be an entire book written about supporting drainage, but we'll have to keep it at high level here. The first thing you can and should do is identify whether you're experiencing the impacts of sluggish drainage in any of the systems designed to support it. Some of the signs of poor drainage are incredibly simple to identify; others are difficult to interpret without the help of lab testing.

Take a quick inventory of these symptoms. How many apply to you?

- Pooping less than once per day
- Inability to sweat
- Puffy feet or ankles
- Bloating after eating
- Skin issues/reaction
- Brain fog
- Fatigue

That's not an exhaustive list, but it might give you an idea of whether drainage is a problem for you right now. As with cellular energy, we're not passing "Go" or collecting $200 until we solve this one. Your body will not make significant progress toward healing until its drainage is working properly.

There are numerous tactics that you can try to support each individual system. Describing them all would take more space than we have available, but here are some ideas you can quickly implement, as well as a quick description of who might benefit the most from trying them.

By the way, you don't want to hear it again and I don't want to say it again, but proper hydration is critical for drainage as well. You can't outmaneuver a dehydrated system. Drink water, a lot of it, if you're serious about making progress against any of the symptoms of perimenopause.

Supporting Drainage So You Can Thrive
The Gut

The gut is the linchpin in the drainage conversation. Everyone should take the time to support their gut, but this is especially important if you're experiencing bloating, fatigue, constipation, or even just pooping less often than once per day.

Here are some key tactics for supporting the gut:

Castor Oil Packs: At the time I'm writing this, castor oil packs are really enjoying a moment on social media. But my patients have been using them for years. Many of them report that they are of major benefit to the gut. The essence of a castor oil pack is soaking a cloth in castor oil and applying it directly over the area of interest. In this case, that would be your gut. There are many great instructional guides for applying castor oil packs correctly, and I encourage you to make use of those resources before trying this.

Supplementation: Don't misread this—we are specifically talking about supplemental support, not laxatives. If you're reliant on laxatives, you're not supporting your body's natural process, but essentially putting a Band-Aid on a problem. A good-quality supplement *supports* normal bowel function.

A number of herbal ingredients can help the stool absorb more water, and support the digestive and elimination process in doing so. Look for supplements incorporating such ingredients as aloe vera leaf, wormwood, black walnut, garlic bulb, and clove bud. I'm okay with the use of senna leaf (one you may be familiar with) as well, when incorporated in moderation.

Physical Activity: Movement supports bowel function. Even a brisk walk is a great aid in this.

Abdominal Self-Massage: Look up some techniques for this. You may find that doing this regularly helps stimulate the bowels.

Liver & Kidneys

Whereas the liver relies on the gut to drain, kidneys drain primarily through urination. Both of these organs are critical and oftentimes stressed.

Hydration & Nutrition: Both of these are especially important for the kidneys and liver. Read earlier in this chapter for more information on these topics.

Limit Toxin Exposure: This is a can of worms. For now, we'll just crack it open. Your liver filters toxins out of your blood, and the more you tax it, the harder it has to work. Alcohol is one toxin many people dump into their body on a daily basis. You may need to seriously reconsider this, if you hope to heal. Other toxins aren't as blatantly introduced to the bloodstream. Yet we breathe them in or consume them daily—toxins from food, environment, or household products. We'll get into some easy swaps later on, but just know that many of these swaps will support drainage by reducing your toxic load.

Supplementation: Powerful supplements exist for kidney and liver support. My absolute favorite is a good-quality tauroursodeoxycholic acid (TUDCA). This can be an absolute game changer for many people. NAC and ALA both offer great benefits for the liver as well. Conveniently, there's overlap here with cellular energy supplementation. I'm also a fan of a good-quality milk thistle supplement. You can even find a number of milk thistle teas on the market, if you'd rather go that route. For specific supplement recommendations, see the Resources section (page 185).

Lymphatic & Glymphatic Systems

The lymphatic system is kind of like the body's oil filter, and the glymphatic system is the brain's equivalent of the lymphatic system. Both of these systems seek to eliminate waste and toxins from the body.

Lymphatic Massage & Dry Brushing: Lymphatic massage is a specific form of massage, and you can sometimes find massage therapists who are specialized in it. Self-massage can also be done at home, following proper techniques. The end goal is to stimulate your lymphatic system to promote normal function. Dry brushing works to the same end. In this case, you take a soft brush to your skin and brush gently toward your heart, to promote lymph flow.

Movement: This is a theme in the drainage conversation. Physical activity stimulates lymphatic drainage as well.

Sleep: We've already had the sleep talk, but believe it or not, good sleep is an essential for drainage as well. Your glymphatic system is especially known to do its best work, "cleaning out" the brain, as you sleep. You can help it by improving your quality of sleep, having your last bite of food three hours before bedtime, and prioritizing sleep whenever possible.

Sweat Glands & Respiratory System

We're at the end of our drainage crash course, with perhaps the two most overlooked systems participating. Your sweat glands do an excellent job of filtering out toxins when they're working properly, and your respiratory system literally filters them out of your body 24/7.

Avoid Antiperspirants: No one likes to stink. No one likes to sweat. However, when you block your sweat glands from doing the work they were designed to do, there are consequences. Antiperspirants inhibit a natural process that, in part, filters toxins out of your body. By restraining them from doing this job, you're essentially choosing to retain those toxins.

You can wear deodorant to combat body odor, but I strongly encourage you to select a deodorant that is merely that—NOT an antiperspirant. The more natural your selection, the better. Especially if hormone health is a concern, look for aluminum-free deodorants. I get it; some argue that natural deodorants don't work as well and they can't afford the sacrifice. If this is the case for you, consider switching to natural options when you can afford to, and relegate the other stuff to an as-needed basis—big events and the like.

Sweat, If You Can: Once the antiperspirant is out of the way, I encourage you to sweat appropriately. To me, this means that when you're active on a warm day, you should sweat. When you're sitting on the couch with the A/C on and still sweating? That might be excessive. And yet, some people don't sweat appropriately. Over the years I've had numerous patients tell me, "Dr. Greg, I don't sweat. I swell."

Does that sound like you? Reddened, swollen skin without a drop of sweat? Or does the most strenuous exercise leave you barely glistening? That's a drainage issue! All of the action items here can help open up those drainage pathways to make sweating possible again.

Nebulizing: Earlier, we talked about breathwork. Your respiratory system is already pumping hard to filter toxins out of your body, and you don't even think about it. But sometimes, it pays to give the respiratory system some backup. That's where nebulizing comes in. A nebulizer is a tool that vaporizes liquid so that it can be inhaled through a nasal or an oral breath. If that sounds like a fancy piece of medical machinery, you can actually purchase one online for well under $100.

When nebulizing, it's a great time to practice the box breathing tactic we learned on page 28 (take deep breaths, hold them in, and then slowly let them out), alternating between oral and nasal breaths.

Drainage Troubleshooting

If you try some of these tactics and still find that your drainage is sluggish, that's okay, but don't press on and try to ignore it. Sometimes, deeper drainage work becomes a necessity. That might not sound ideal, but at least you're getting answers about why you feel the way that you do. A natural healing process can take time, and everyone's journey is different.

2.

THE JOURNEY YOU'RE TAKING: UNDERSTANDING HORMONES

You may have skipped straight to this chapter, and I don't blame you. The hormone conversation is on every woman's mind at this time in her life, and the answers they're given aren't clear. By the way, I hope you do go back and read the first chapter, because addressing hormones without first addressing energy and drainage will get you nowhere. But that said, a hormonal shift was clearly the catalyst for many who feel as if they were moving along fine before the wheels suddenly came off.

I want us to back up the truck and take a look under the hood together. You've probably been given a lot of advice about what you should do to address hormonal shifts and imbalances, but has anyone ever paused to have a conversation about the hormones themselves? Many women go through their lives hearing phrases like "estrogen dominance" or "hormone imbalance" without getting a thorough enough picture of what the implications are. We tend to know different hormonal states and conditions by their symptoms, rather than the functions of each hormone.

Why do we even need to understand the functions? Because the moment we do, the pieces start coming together. The *why* behind each symptom is more important than the symptom itself, and if you dive into the function of each hormone, you can begin to understand why you feel the way you feel.

Grasping the Hormone Cascade

Before we dive into the specific hormones that impact the way you feel and function, it's important to have a high level of understanding of where these hormones come from. A little-known fact is that all hormones originate from the same root before trickling down like a waterfall into the different forms that we're familiar with.

Let's go to the river at the top of the waterfall. Before any hormones are created by the body, they begin at the source—cholesterol. That's right, all of your hormones come from cholesterol. Although villainized, cholesterol is essential to the body, when in balance. Without cholesterol, there would be no testosterone, estrogen, or progesterone.

As cholesterol begins to trickle down the waterfall, critical factors come into play. Two worth pointing out are the thyroid's role in the process, as well as vitamin A. Complex processes unfold that allow the body to efficiently and effectively convert cholesterol into the hormones you need. A vitamin A deficiency or a dysfunctional thyroid will only stand in the way.

With the help of these processes and others, cholesterol triggers the release of new hormones in the body. The first in line is pregnenolone. Pregnenolone is the mother hormone that others originate from. As a stand-alone, this hormone makes a positive impact on cognitive health and other bodily functions. However, in the perimenopause conversation, it is primarily of interest as a precursor to the key hormones that are impacted during this phase of life.

To avoid confusion, we won't cover the entire hormone cascade. But a summary is that the trickle-down effect continues as pregnenolone triggers two completely different kinds of hormones to be created: dehydroepiandrosterone (DHEA) and progesterone. On the DHEA side, we have such hormones as testosterone and estrogen. The progesterone side produces progesterone and cortisol.

Meet the Hormones

If you have some knowledge on the topic of hormone health, three hormones probably come to mind when you consider where this chapter will go. What I have to tell you is that those three hormones aren't even the most impactful of the eight types we're actually going to discuss. However, these first three—the sex hormones—do play an important role, and since estrogen, progesterone, and testosterone are likely the top three known to most of us, let's talk about them before we introduce the next five hormones that have seats at the table. As we discuss each hormone, we'll especially focus on the role they play in perimenopause.

Estrogen

Estrogen needs a new PR rep, because it's earned a bad name. This is the hormone that's dominant in the follicular and ovulatory phases of your cycle. By the way, let's pause there. Do you know whether/when you ovulate?

My parents used to go around and teach something called natural family planning, when I was growing up. Natural family planning relies on the ability to identify ovulation when it is beginning, but that skill set can be valuable beyond family planning. If you're not familiar with it, learn the signs that let you know that your body is entering the ovulatory phase. Temperature, mucus, and even cervix position can all attest to whether your body is ovulating. It matters because, if you're not experiencing the ovulatory phase, that alone gives many clues about where you are in your journey.

Bad reputation aside, estrogen should really be looked at as your gas pedal. In the estrogen dominant stages of your menstrual cycle, you should feel energized and ready to take on challenges.

This would be the time in your cycle where you can take on higher-intensity workouts, lift heavy weights, or just get things done, in general. By the way, estrogen is responsible for such things as skin health, brain health, and tissue elasticity. When in balance, it's not the villain!

Progesterone

If estrogen is the gas pedal, progesterone is the brake pedal. Progesterone allows the body to, in a sense, chill out. After reading that, you might not be surprised to know that progesterone is the number one hormone I find to be deficient during perimenopause. Many women come into my clinic feeling that they're all gas and no brake.

So, what happens when you're all gas and no brake? Get ready, because if this is you, these signs will be easily identifiable:

- Anxiety
- Emotional instability
- Not sleeping well
- Shortened second half of your cycle

Sound like you at all? Progesterone is a profoundly important hormone to have in balance. If estrogen's left to run rampant without the balance from progesterone, things go haywire. We'll continue the progesterone conversation shortly.

Testosterone

The final sex hormone in the trio is testosterone. This hormone is very commonly deficient even before perimenopause. Many people think of testosterone as spurring aggression, libido, and sex drive. Although it does play a role in each of those areas, there's actually a much more telltale sign that you're experiencing testosterone deficiency or insufficiency. Have you ever found yourself sitting on the couch with a pile of responsibilities and not one fiber of your being can find any motivation to tackle them?

Oftentimes, testosterone is responsible—in men and women—for a complete lack of motivation. We can all be lazy once in a while, regardless of testosterone levels, but if you've found yourself consistently lacking motivation to get up and tackle tasks you used to care about, you may be testosterone deficient!

Cortisol

Now that we're all on the same page about the sex hormones, it's time to move past them and into the other four that really matter in perimenopause. If you've been online or grabbed a book like this one during the past couple of years, you can attest to the fact that a lot of conversation happens around this hormone called cortisol. Unfortunately, there's a lot of conversation, but not a lot of understanding.

Cortisol has an association with tiny organs called your adrenal glands. Your adrenal glands, which sit on top of your kidneys, are designed to respond to stress. By the way, that's a good thing! We need to have the capacity to respond to stress. What we're not designed to do is respond to continual stress over long periods of time that never backs down or cools off. If your body has this sense that it's always running for its life, that's not healthy.

Now, cortisol is a hormone that fluctuates substantially over the course of a single day. In the morning, something called a cortisol awakening response causes your cortisol level to rise by 50 to 160 percent within 30 minutes of waking up. So, if your cortisol levels are optimal, you should wake up in a state of relaxation and then be "game on" within that next half-hour. I'll take a guess right now that you might say, "There's no game on." If so, we'll get to that!

But for now, let's assume the cortisol awakening response functions optimally. What's next? Like a bell curve, cortisol levels will now slowly decline throughout the rest of the day. Ideally, by the time you're ready for bed, cortisol levels will be at or near their absolute lowest for the day, so you can enjoy a time of rest.

You might be wondering now whether your body missed the part where the cortisol levels are supposed to ramp up and then *actually come down*. We'll cover that as well, in a bit.

Melatonin

If we're honest, most of us think of melatonin as a sleep aid or a supplement. Depending on which expert you've been listening to, you either consider a melatonin supplement a powerful asset or perhaps a crutch with some dangerous side effects. But let's put the supplement aside for a minute—melatonin is actually a hormone naturally produced by your body. When in balance, melatonin allows your body to achieve deep, restful sleep. It's this kind of sleep that allows your body to recycle and rejuvenate.

This could be said at any point during the hormone fly-through, but it's especially relevant with melatonin, since so many people supplement it: You have to picture hormones as a symphony orchestra. In concert with other instruments, the trombone sounds great, but if the trombone stages a takeover and you're inundated with the blasts of it as it powers over all other instruments, the whole orchestra sounds off.

Hormone levels don't need to be high enough; they need to be in balance with all of the others. If they aren't, you can experience the very real effects of too much of a good thing. Don't think for a moment that you can just flood your body with enough of one thing to create a solution to an issue. This isn't a specific opinion on using melatonin as a sleep aid, just an important reminder to consider all of the essential hormones as working together to perform as a symphony. Band-Aid solutions may provide a quick fix, but we can't go on too long patching bullet wounds with Band-Aids, so be careful of thinking of this one as solved.

Vitamin D

Yes, you read that right. Vitamin D is the peculiar name we've given this hormone that we're all familiar with but don't consider to be a hormone. Believe it or not, though, vitamin D really is a hormone. And not only that, it's one of the most interesting and essential hormones. I have for years observed it to be among the most commonly deficient hormones I see in lab results. One 2011 study found that 42 percent of the population is vitamin D deficient [8]. Oh, and by the way, that's considering a conventional reference range.

As we had discussed earlier, conventional lab test reference ranges are based on large sample sizes of an entire population that is not well. If we were to consider vitamin D deficiency as anything less than the optimal level, we'd likely see that an outrageously high percentage of the population falls short of that raised bar.

So, why does it matter? In my postdoctoral work with World-Link Medical Academy, vitamin D was easily one of the most discussed hormones. No one should be pushing it to the side in any perimenopause conversation. Vitamin D provides critical support to the adrenal glands, the immune system, and, by the way, energy production.

I will tell you anecdotally that the number one thing my clients report after getting their vitamin D levels up is having more energy. Vitamin D is massively important for this. It's also a key factor in mood regulation. If you've found yourself in a gloomier state, you might consider taking steps to support your vitamin D levels.

Keep in mind that vitamin D is fat-soluble. It can only be digested if it's in a fat state. We'll talk more later on about how to absorb vitamin D, but if you're already sold on picking up a supplement, just ensure that it provides the delivery system that takes this into account. By the way, a good vitamin D supplement will typically include vitamin K_2 as well.

Insulin

If your hormones are playing in a symphony, insulin has one of the first chairs. This is one of the most essential pieces in the puzzle that's often overlooked. A lot of people are familiar with insulin and its association with diabetes or the term "insulin resistance." Insulin resistance crops up when the body is barraged by stress or the standard American diet (also known as S.A.D.).

After a major glucose response, you have glucose in your body. Glucose relies on insulin to come alongside it, and insulin has to get inside your cells. That process should then play out and this could be the end of the story. But for those who are insulin resistant, what's actually happening is that the cells are not letting insulin in. Many people get this confused, but it's not insulin's fault! The cells are, themselves, resistant to taking in the insulin.

There are actually 10 different hijackers of hormone receptivity. If they've been hijacked, hormones can't be received as easily as they should be. One of the clearest ways we see this is in the case of insulin resistance, but it's applicable across all of the hormones. This is where a lot of hormone clinics go wrong. Rather than addressing hormone receptivity, they continue to dump more and more hormones into the body.

Picture a car that needs gas. Pumping in hormones without addressing hormone receptivity is like taking the nozzle of the gas pump and spraying the gas all over your car. Maybe a few drops get into the tank due to the sheer volume, but almost all of your work "fueling" your car will be wasted as it fails to ever enter the tank. If you want to see the benefits of hormone therapy, you have to work on hormone receptivity and evict the hijackers.

Insulin is highly regulatory when it comes to the stress of your system. If your system is stressed, there's a cortisol imbalance, and a cortisol imbalance can easily trigger insulin resistance. At this point, all your body is trying to do is survive. By the way, I want to let you know that it's not just your diet that can cause insulin resistance, because that's probably what you've been told. There's more at play here sometimes. Such conditions as polycystic ovarian syndrome (PCOS) can also cause insulin resistance.

Thyroid Hormones

Last, but certainly not least, are thyroid hormones. A lot of women become all too familiar with them, due to struggles with hypothyroidism, hyperthyroidism, Graves' disease, or Hashimoto's thyroiditis. For most women, their doctor is interested in running one test for a specific marker called thyroid stimulating hormone (TSH).

This is not actually a bioavailable hormone in the body. It does not increase metabolism when optimal. In reality, TSH is actually a neurological hormone that tells your brain to release more of another thyroid hormone—one called T4.

If your TSH is too high, what your body is really doing is saying, "We need more T4!" T4—free T4, specifically—is like crude oil. Crude oil needs to be refined into gasoline to be usable in your car's engine. Similarly, free T4 needs to be converted into free T3 to be usable in the body. By the way, 80 percent of that conversion happens within the liver and the gut . . . remember our conversations about optimal liver and gut health?

The thyroid hormones are massively important in perimenopause, and an unbelievable number of women who come to me are experiencing the symptoms of a suboptimally functioning thyroid, whether they know it or not. Do any of these symptoms sound familiar?

- Weight-loss resistance (a big one!)
- Fatigue
- Dry skin
- Dry hair
- Constipation
- Thinning of the lateral third of the eyebrow
- Brittle nails
- Fertility issues
- Period issues

Wow, what a list, right? By the way, your lab test results don't have to be outside a medical reference range for your thyroid to be functioning at a less-than-optimal capacity.

The Symphony: Finding Hormone Balance

You made it through the hormone fly-through and met eight key musicians in the symphony. Thinking of addressing each of those areas independent of one another sounds complex, doesn't it? You're already taking a mental inventory of where to put all the supplements and how to find the time to fit in all the lifestyle hacks.

The good and bad news is that a symphony works as one unit. We can simplify this conversation to talk about two things that really define the phrase we know of as "hormone balance": ratio and rhythm. *Ratio* determines how much each individual instrument is featured and at what places within the music. *Rhythm* simply asks whether we're all playing the same music and everyone is on beat.

You can probably understand the significance of how the hormones interact. Too much progesterone in one part of your cycle could mean you don't ovulate, but too much estrogen could mean estrogen dominance. Everything exists within a very fine balance. Let's use insulin as another example. If you eat a meal that's heavy in carbohydrates, we *want* an insulin response to happen. If you're eating heavy protein and healthy fats without any carbs, we *don't* want that response. It's not about having enough of something, it's about the right instruments playing at the right time.

By the way, some of the hormones (testosterone, for instance) are fairly consistent and level. Not all of them are swinging up and down! But because of those that do fluctuate, it's very difficult to run a single set of lab tests and get an exact picture of whether you are experiencing hormone imbalance. There are absolutely standards to aim for in some sense, and there are targets to pursue, but there are many ingredients to be mindful of.

For instance, it should be strongly considered where you're at in the menstrual cycle on the day the lab testing is done. The person evaluating the testing results should be able to understand that phase of the cycle to the extent that the results are analyzed in light of it. Keep in mind that biochemical individuality is also at play, so even the idea of where things "should be" can vary to an extent. I hope I don't sound as if I'm downplaying the significance of lab testing—it is an amazing tool! But no tool spits out a perfect game plan. Lab tests can point us in the right direction, but just because test results look "good" doesn't mean you feel good.

Let's go back to that idea of building the right supplements or medicine cabinet. I want you to know before reading on that this really isn't as simple as relating to some symptoms and grabbing some vitamins to address those symptoms. The era of social media and the many success stories shared there have trained us to think of medicine as *this for that*.

I've been Western medicine's critic on a *this for that* approach at times. I don't like the concept of presenting a symptom and matching it to a prescription. But here's what I also need to clarify: Some of these natural health doctors and influencers criticize that method and then present the same exact thing! You can't simply replace a medication with a supplement and follow the same exact *this for that* technique. It's not that simple, and you're going to end up wasting hundreds or thousands of dollars on supplements that don't work.

Revisiting the Foundational Systems

If this book convinces you of anything, I hope it's that hormones don't operate inside a vacuum. If solving a crazy perimenopause (and eventually menopause) roller coaster ride were so simple, hormone clinics would have cracked the code by now. We'd slap everyone onto a hormone protocol and be done with it. Remember how, earlier in the book, I mentioned that there are cultures that don't view perimenopause and menopause the same way we do? You might also recall that I mentioned a significant portion of women go through these phases symptom-free, or close to it.

This has to be about more than just hormones. And if we understand how the body functions, I think we can explain why that is. We've already talked extensively about the nervous system, proper drainage, and cellular energy. But don't let go of these as the more "advanced" information comes into play. They matter, and I believe failure to address these facets of the journey lead us to frustration and failure.

Nothing happens without cellular energy; healing is stalled if the nervous system doesn't allow it; and drainage equips you to keep going. Hold on to that.

The Perimenopause Hormone Ripple Effect

Okay, let's look at a practical example of what goes down inside the body during perimenopause. Every woman is different, so this exact scenario may or may not encompass what you're experiencing. More important than being accurate to your circumstances, I want to demonstrate how all of the hormones and systems we've covered can interact with one another. A domino effect is at play, and if we can map that out, we can succeed in addressing the symptoms that result from it. Having each of the players in our symphony in mind, we can better understand how one hormone isn't just high or low, but how an entire chain reaction can be set off.

Let's use a fictional character by the name of Ellen for this example. Ellen was going through her life as usual when, all of a sudden, it seemed that the wheels came off as she came into perimenopause. Ellen, like many women in perimenopause, feels as if she's all gas and no brake. Her body's always ramped, and she has no ability to really rest. She's irritable, experiencing mood swings, gaining weight, and getting hot flashes. She can't sleep, her head is always hurting, and she experiences fatigue as a result of all of the above.

Ellen's not just imagining things: She really is all gas and no brakes—she's progesterone deficient and her estrogen is running the show. We've covered this example a little bit already, but let's carry this farther than we have previously, so we can understand how the other hormones come into play.

Since Ellen's dealing with low progesterone, cortisol is left to go on a wild goose chase. It goes on a rampage, and suddenly Ellen feels as if she needs to be figuratively looking over her shoulder for the next threat. She's gaining weight in her belly and on her face, and her muscles seem weakened. But, oh, by the way, another component comes into play in this chain reaction—her nervous system is actually shifted into the fight-or-flight state.

Now, Ellen's in a real state of stress. Her digestion is slowing, she's becoming constipated, and a constant sense of anxiousness makes her heart beat faster even when it shouldn't.

Whew. Sound familiar? We're not done yet. This whole cascade of reactions actually leads to decreased immune function, and that pulls another hormone, vitamin D, into the equation. Due to the many factors in this scenario, vitamin D is now reducing as well. That opens Ellen up to the threats of chronic infection and toxicity.

What a journey, right? By the way, we moved past estrogen pretty quickly in this example. For most women, it is declining during perimenopause as well, and a host of symptoms come as a result of that. Many of the symptoms of low estrogen actually overlap with the symptoms of low progesterone—mood changes, irritability, hot flashes, fatigue, trouble sleeping . . . It's possible to experience the effects of low estrogen during perimenopause, but it's also important to note that we can't forget about the hormones' relationship to one another. Just because your estrogen is also low doesn't mean that your body isn't estrogen dominant. That depends on the balance between progesterone and estrogen, rather than just the amount of each independently.

Meet the Villain: Endocrine-Disrupting Chemicals

The term "endocrine disrupter" is gaining some steam in recent years, as people are becoming more aware of the concept. An endocrine-disrupting chemical is named appropriately. These chemicals have the ability to actually disrupt the optimal function of your endocrine systems. They can hijack your body and impact hormone receptivity by essentially masquerading as a hormone your body needs to function.

There are now tests that can measure the presence of endocrine-disrupting chemicals in the body.

So, what are endocrine-disrupting chemicals?
- Plastics
- Phthalates
- Per- and polyfluoroalkyl substances (PFAs), a.k.a. forever chemicals
- Heavy metals
- Pesticides
- Herbicides
- Flame retardants

At a glance, this might look like a list of things you wouldn't come into contact with on a regular basis. On the contrary, almost all of us live in homes full of products containing endocrine-disrupting chemicals. We interact with them on a daily basis—sometimes in microdoses and sometimes in larger capacities than we'd be comfortable with knowing about.

Here are some common household products that are likely to contain one or more of these endocrine-disrupting chemicals.
- Candles
- Air fresheners
- Living room chairs & sofas
- Carpet
- Cleaning supplies
- Hand & dish soaps
- Lotions
- Makeup
- Shampoo & deodorant
- Processed food

Unfortunately, the list goes on. Many times, even more natural-looking brands will incorporate one or more of these endocrine-disrupting chemicals into their products. What's the danger here? Believe it or not, these chemicals actually have the ability to steal a hormone's ability to bind to your cells. They mimic hormones closely enough that they can dock in place of a hormone.

Let's use insulin as an example to understand how this plays out. Your cells need insulin, but the binding sites on your cells are occupied by endocrine-disrupting chemicals. Your nervous system, noticing the lack of insulin in the cells, sends the message, "We need more insulin!" This triggers insulin production. Now, as your cells are insulin resistant, there becomes a blunting of insulin receptors throughout your entire body.

Because insulin is so intimately intertwined with the sex hormones, this can set off a chain reaction. In the end, your body, identifying itself as in a state of chronic stress, could actually shift away from being in a place of fertility and thus optimal menstrual cycles. It is instead prone to shift attention to immune system support—producing white blood cells, platelets, and more. In the end, your hormones are out of balance.

So, what does a hormone clinic or a doctor do when a woman comes to them with hormones out of balance? They try to balance the hormones! But what if the woman's body shifted into this defensive state intelligently? What if, instead of throwing in hormones to arm wrestle the body's natural response, we actually paused to appreciate it and understand that something might indeed be going on that needs addressing?

In the case of endocrine-disrupting chemicals, there really is no better solution than to swap them out! By limiting your body's intake, you can aid hormone receptivity tremendously. It might take time for your body to shift back into an optimal state, but the long-term support will go a long way.

Top Products to Swap Out

I'm a realistic kind of person. Let me be the first to tell you that if you go too far down the endocrine-disruptor rabbit hole, you'll be more confused than when you first entered. You might come to a disturbing realization that practically everything seems to contain endocrine-disrupting chemicals (EDCs). I encourage you to follow your gut when it comes to making healthy swaps, but it's important not to obsess over it. An unhealthy obsession runs the risk of creating just as much stress as the EDCs did in the first place!

Yes, many products contain EDCs. No, you will never fully eliminate your exposure to them. You don't need to become the person who can't eat dinner at a friend's house due to their dish soap, but you can take steps to control what you can control.

To again use the rain barrel example, toxic load is like one that's filled to the brim and ready to overflow. The more water you can remove, the farther you get from overflow even if the bucket's not completely empty. Make the responsible swaps and trust your body to handle the rest.

By the way, making these swaps can be done affordably, but it can be costly to throw out entire cabinets of product and replace them all at once. My recommendation is to replace each item as the last bottle of the previous version empties out. Instead of buying the same hand soap you always do, simply purchase a purer product on your next visit to the store!

But when you do make those swaps, what are you looking for, exactly? It can be very time-consuming and frustrating to stand in an aisle, reading entire ingredient labels full of alphabet soup ingredients. If you start by seeking out just the single word "fragrance," it will go a long way. This garbage-basket term allows brands to select from almost 2,000 different chemicals and essentially rebrand them under this one neat and tidy name—"fragrance." Fragrance is typically chock-full of phthalates and other nasty things. A lot of brands have caught on and like to use phrases like this one: "Fragranced *with* natural fragrances." Notice the word *with* doesn't necessarily imply the absence of artificial fragrance—only the presence of some amount of natural fragrance.

As relates to food, I'd advise making reasonable swaps that move you away from heavy herbicide and pesticide consumption. Not everyone can afford to eat all organic, and that's okay! If this is you, the Environmental Working Group (EWG)'s "Dirty Dozen" resource can come in handy. If all you can do is swap out these kinds of heavily sprayed produce in favor of their organic versions, that's a win.

So here it is, the Dirty Dozen. And yes, these are in order—the worst of the worst is number 1, but all 12 are among the most pesticide-laden conventionally grown produce in America:

1. Spinach
2. Strawberries
3. Kale, collards, and mustard greens
4. Grapes
5. Peaches

6. Cherries
7. Nectarines
8. Pears
9. Apples
10. Blackberries
11. Blueberries
12. Potatoes

By the way, I know this is a lot to keep track of. They're not paying me a dime to say this, but there are two resources I recommend to everyone. My personal favorite is an app called Yuka. This app allows you to scan a barcode in the grocery store to get an instant analysis of the potential health impacts a product carries. It will give scores from 0 to 100, color-code things as good or bad choices, and provide some breakdowns if you're curious. This is such a helpful resource!

In a similar fashion, the EWG has an online database where you can look up your favorite products to see how they're graded on similar criteria.

I want to emphasize again—the point of bringing awareness to EDCs is not to create your next new obsession. Before you go on a stressful, relentless pursuit to eliminate them all, just take some deep breaths. Change what you can change, and don't panic over the rest.

How Hormone Imbalance Impacts the Rest of Your Body

Hormone imbalance is famous for the symptoms it can cause. We've explored already how such things as high or low estrogen, progesterone, insulin, vitamin D, and more bring a slug of symptoms along with them. But there's another important part of the conversation, one that's often skipped: how hormone imbalance affects all the other systems in your body.

Sometimes, a deficiency in a hormone doesn't itself create the symptoms you experience. Instead, the impact of imbalanced hormones causes stress on another system, and that system creates the symptoms. We could spend the rest of the book diving in on this topic, but I want to explore the one organ that matters most in this conversation: the liver!

The liver is undoubtedly the most overworked, underpaid organ: Every few minutes, it filters every drop of blood in your entire body. Another thing the liver does, interestingly enough, is shuttle estrogen and progesterone throughout your body at ovulation, and then again during menstruation. So, if your whole cycle is imbalanced, we should look to the liver as well, since it's playing this essential role.

The liver has many roles, and because of that, too much stress can make it feel tapped. Things start falling off its plate. So, what does the liver do? First of all, it has a huge digestive role. It produces a fat emulsifier called bile, which essentially breaks down fat. Think of dish soap breaking down the fats stuck to a plate. By the way, you might be familiar with a little organ called the gallbladder, as it relates to bile.

Many adults have had their gallbladder removed. I want you to know that many of my colleagues and I have observed a correlation between gallbladder removal and a stressed liver. So, if you've had yours out, you may want to take the time to ensure your liver is getting some extra love. There's absolutely hope for you, and this is nothing to panic about. If you give the extra time and attention to your liver, you'll do just fine.

What are some other roles the liver plays? We've actually already discussed one, but the liver is responsible for the lion's share of thyroid hormone conversion. So, if you're keeping track, we've already addressed that estrogen, progesterone, and thyroid hormones are all dependent on the liver to function optimally.

By the way, we just glazed over it quickly, but I want to come back to how your liver filters every drop of blood in your body every few minutes. Think of every infection, toxin, chemical, or other matter that has ever entered your body. Doesn't filtering through all of that seem like a big job? The more you fill that proverbial rain barrel, the more the liver is forced to focus resources on this essential task so you can survive! So, if you then demand your liver to focus on shuttling the sex hormones through your body, it might just tell you no!

To illustrate my point, I'm just going to be completely honest for a moment. Some of the toughest clinical cases I have seen have been women who have intervened to move their body into fertility via prescriptions or other modern methodologies, such as in vitro fertilization (IVF). I'm grateful for fertility and for babies, but the fact remains that sometimes, the body prevented fertility for a reason, and when we force it into fertility without addressing the root cause, it can spell trouble.

Where's the Hormone Therapy Talk?!

Alright, we dug in deep during this chapter before ever getting to the conversation surrounding hormone replacement therapy (HRT). First things first: I want to distinguish the reality that hormone therapy isn't one singular approach, as you may have been led to believe. There are actually numerous ways to approach hormone therapy. The avenues you're likely thinking of are prescribed, but others utilize natural products sold over the counter.

The most important distinction here is between bioidentical and synthetic hormones. If you've ever heard about some of the nasty research that's been done on hormone replacement therapy, it's the synthetic hormone conversation—I can almost guarantee it. Synthetic hormones were the ones utilized in disastrous, flawed studies that became famous in the 1990s. Synthetic hormones have been meaningfully tied to various forms of cancer and heart disease—that's why you'll be asked by your health-care practitioner whether you have a family history of either.

I would be very hesitant to ever be comfortable with anyone being on any synthetic hormone. That said, look at how many women are on birth control; perhaps you're one of them. This is an example of one long-standing, legacy product that's only now starting to take some heat for the unintended side effects. A full dissection of birth control is outside the scope of this book, but I do feel strongly that birth control has gone in and ravaged many women's bodies without taking the blame for it.

By the way, I'm not against family planning, but it needs to be acknowledged that being on a synthetic hormone for years or decades may have unintended side effects. When you come in and intervene with a very fragile, very intricate system for an extended period of time, you run some risks. Having just read about this, you might be taking an inventory right now, wondering whether the damage done could be insurmountable.

Here's what I want you to know: The body is designed to heal. The body always aims to return to a state of homeostasis, where everything's in balance. If you have used synthetic hormones, you are not irreparably damaged; however, you might have some work to do.

So, if synthetic hormones aren't the answer, what is? Bioidentical hormones are an option gaining increasing popularity. These hormones are literally named for being practically identical to the real hormones found within the human body. They aren't a substitute for the real thing—they can essentially function as the real thing. Bioidentical hormones are typically sourced from such plants as wild yams and soy. The compounds are extracted, chemically converted, and then checked for purity.

You may have seen supplemental products, such as Mexican wild yam tinctures or creams, but these products can also be put to use by compounding pharmacies to create prescribed hormone treatments similar to their synthetic counterparts.

Now, I am a fan of bioidentical hormone therapy (BHRT) when used appropriately. Although it might be tempting to try this as an "Easy" button, I continue to stand by my opinion that it won't work for the long haul without support. It brings us back to the example of dumping gasoline all over a car without getting anything in the tank. Many hormone clinics will happily show you success stories while pushing under the rug others that were a less-than-optimal experience.

Do you have cellular energy, your drainage is optimal, your nervous system is settled, and your liver is functioning? At that point, you're primed to see the results from BHRT. Now, before you drive to the clinic, I need to make you aware of one other and perhaps lesser-known option for hormone replenishment and restoration. So, stay tuned for that, but before we go there, I also want to make you aware of the one hormone I actually do not advise taking . . . and it's probably not what you'd expect!

Why I Don't Encourage Estradiol

In most circumstances, I don't encourage women in perimenopause to consider taking estradiol. It might sound counterintuitive, but part of the goal of perimenopause is to help the ovaries make a smooth transition into menopause. I hate the terminology behind it, but conventional medicine would refer to this as the "failing" of the ovaries. By the way, this goal aside, I find that this is rarely ever a hormone that there's not enough of already.

You've already heard me talk a bit about the concept of estrogen running the show. A more formal label for that is "estrogen dominance." Many women in perimenopause are estrogen dominant, and taking more estrogen sure isn't going to solve that problem.

Making Your Hormones Work for You

You're ready to get off the roller coaster and reclaim the old you. If that's going to happen, you'll have to optimize your hormones. When optimized and in harmony, your hormones are a wonderful gift that promote health and well-being.

Progesterone

If estrogen is left practically untouched, what's optimized? Many hormones can be optimized, but progesterone is a significant one. When women have their progesterone optimized, it's almost as if they can finally take a deep breath after a long time. The ability to rest and digest is restored.

The tricky thing about progesterone optimization is that, while lab testing should be considered, no single "gold standard," definite number in the tests tells us you've reached an optimal state. So lab testing, then, is only part of the analysis. The other end is hearing from women like yourself about how they're actually feeling. As a woman, you are intuitive! Trust yourself to know where you stand.

When you're optimizing progesterone ask yourself:

- Do I feel more like myself?
- Can I relax better?
- Am I sleeping better?
- Am I less edgy?
- Can I wind down in the evenings?

Progesterone optimization can be achieved through prescription BHRT or with the use of natural products you can buy over the counter. We'll discuss those options in depth in future chapters.

Testosterone

If you're low in testosterone, you're likely lacking energy, vitality, and even the metabolic activity that supports weight loss. Testosterone in balance is an amazing thing! That said, you're probably familiar with some of the horror stories about too much testosterone, and we should be mindful of that as well. It presents with such symptoms as oily skin and unwanted hair growth.

By the way, that's why we have to remember in the hormone replenishment world that if a little is good, a lot does not equal better. These are conversations about microdosing—making tiny adjustments rather than huge shifts.

I want to make this clear on the front end—testosterone is a controlled substance. If you want to take testosterone directly, you will need a prescription. However, we've also found in research that hormones that serve as precursors to testosterone can be taken and lead to very good results. These hormones include pregnenolone and DHEA. So long as these hormones (often taken in the form of a supplement) are delivered in a highly bioavailable way, they convert to testosterone very well.

In some cases, it might make sense to skip the prescriptions, compounding pharmacies, and physicians. But the decision is yours. Chapter 4 will help you make that decision.

Thyroid Hormones

When you go to your doctor and the two of you mutually agree that your thyroid hormones should be optimized, there's a good chance you'll walk away with a prescription for something that's essentially built on a basis of desiccated thyroid. The source? Pigs—at least in many cases. So, essentially, a pig thyroid has been dried out and purified, and you are utilizing it to help optimize your thyroid.

In the world of natural supplements, we have access to a similar product. However, in this circumstance, we can utilize a grass-fed, organic beef thyroid. This is an over-the-counter product, and I like it for the ability to control the source and quality of what you're putting into your body. In very pure forms, desiccated thyroid can help provide those T3 and T4 hormones that your body may desperately need.

When we provide this, we see such results as disappearing fatigue, improving metabolism, reduced hair loss, and stronger nails. Oh, and by the way—normal bowel movements!

Maybe you can start to see the balance here. Testosterone and thyroid hormones add fuel to the fire, but progesterone comes in as the soother. Because of this, you can't just start taking six things at once. If something about them doesn't work, you have no idea why it didn't work. If it did work, you might be stuck taking six products every day for years to come, when in reality you need only a couple of them!

Later, we'll help you build a protocol from the ground up. But let it be said now before it's too late: Don't start everything all at once!

What to Do When Lab Testing Results Don't Match How You Feel

I've run thousands upon thousands of advanced medical lab tests. I'm a huge advocate for proper lab testing, and I believe that more comprehensive tests with greater accuracy should be the standard in the American health system. That said, I want to acknowledge that there can always be misalignment between lab testing results and how you actually feel. You may have had the experience of going to your doctor with health concerns, begging them to run lab tests, and then finding that in the end the results came back normal. Now, we've said this before, but lab results are only as good as the person interpreting them. "In range" on a lab test might be called normal by your doctor, but it isn't the same thing as being optimal.

But, for the sake of this example, let's put that aside. Let's assume that, in your lab test results, your hormones appear perfectly in balance and optimal. What should we do in that case, if you continue to experience hormone-related symptoms? I can't speak for your doctor, but I personally honor the symptom—and you can do the same. We can appreciate biochemical individuality to the fullest extent and accept that optimal numbers on a sheet of paper don't override what you're actually feeling.

I want to be careful not to discard the importance of quality lab testing. Without them, we have no reliable way to get a baseline. Even if you come into optimal ranges without feeling optimal, we can still trust the data as accurate. And with accurate data, we can continue to make informed decisions.

You've been trained that symptoms are subjective, but what you're experiencing is real and you need to honor it. So, what's the action step? You can steal a page from my book—start asking questions and record your answers. It's that simple. It's coming back to the State of the Union exercise introduced on page 24. It might sound simplistic, but a detailed questionnaire is exactly what we use at my clinic at this stage in the journey. When lab test results show a thumbs-up, but you know you don't feel that way, the questionnaire takes precedent and becomes your guiding light as you move forward. We're not discarding the accuracy of the lab test results; we're discarding any preconceived notions about how that result should equate to what you actually feel.

It all comes back to the hormone symphony. A skilled conductor understands what each section should sound like. They can skillfully bring in each at the appropriate time, at the right volume, with the right notes. What we know about hormones is that they impact your mood, mindset, longevity, libido, metabolism, sense of well-being, and even the belief that you're in control of your life.

Take an inventory of how you're feeling! Go back to the State of the Union exercise (page 24). If you skipped it, go back and do it. As your lab test values change, you need to understand where you came from, where you're at, and whether you're seeing the progress you need to see.

Should Anyone Avoid Optimizing Hormones?

Welcome to the most controversial portion of this book. This is a question that has to be asked. And by the way, this book isn't a replacement for speaking with a physician who can work with you on a personal basis. Every situation is unique, so there really aren't too many cases where a blanket yes or no exists. If you're looking for a reliable physician that's in tune with much of what we're discussing in this book, I'd encourage you to seek out someone certified at WorldLink Medical Academy. I've taken WorldLink's certification training, and I resonate with its approach to bioidentical hormone replacement therapy.

That aside, let's discuss some of the potential risk factors. The first is a family history of hormone-sensitive cancers. Some people will call this a red light, whereas others will tell you it's more of a "proceed with caution." I'd urge you to not move forward with a conventional (synthetic) hormone replacement program, as those have been directly tied to hormone-sensitive cancers, as noted earlier. As far as BHRT goes, or even some of the natural products we've discussed, the honest truth is that not enough research has been done to draw direct conclusions.

Be aware of this risk factor and have a conversation with a physician you can trust, before proceeding into anything.

Another risk factor is uncontrolled clotting disorders, such as Factor V Leiden. This may not be a hard stop, but it's absolutely a caution light and an indication that you should speak with a medical professional.

This small section might not capture all of the populations who should approach hormone replenishment with caution, but the final one I will specifically address is those who experience hormonal migraines. Oftentimes, we find that people who are impacted in this way just don't respond as well to hormone replenishment.

Actually, I'll add one that you might not be expecting. If you're someone who is unwilling to address diet, lifestyle, and detoxification . . . this is simply not going to work for you. If you're looking for the "Easy" button, this isn't it. You'll be likely to see dismal results, if any at all. I don't mean to sound harsh, but hormone replenishment is not a fix for a stressful and crappy lifestyle. I just want to be as honest as I can.

Don't Be Scared of Your Hormones

If you just read this chapter and now find yourself feeling confused, that's not my intention. However, I want to acknowledge that anything involving hormones absolutely can be confusing at times. My goal is to help you navigate this to the best of my ability. You may need to consider working one-on-one with a new physician or bringing some of this information into conversations with the one you already have. Or you might feel completely empowered to take this on and ease some things in from an over-the-counter perspective.

Here's my encouragement. Millions upon millions of women take a vitamin D supplement. Millions more are on prescriptions that work toward managing hormones. These range from birth control to thyroid medications and beyond. How many people do you know who actively take melatonin supplements? As many as 2.5 million women today are estimated to be using bioidentical hormone replacement therapy in some regard.

I don't blindly recommend hormone replacement, replenishment, or management. Risk factors exist and some women should speak with their physicians about them. I've been vocal about my disapproval of synthetic hormones. My point is that hormones are powerful and what they can do is powerful. We should approach hormones with respect and caution, but tens of millions of Americans already interact with products brushing up against hormones already, and you probably have as well.

Don't be scared of your hormones or of addressing them with care, caution, and responsibility. A conversation with your doctor might be a great starting place. But fear shouldn't stand in the way of at least weighing your options.

Slow Down & Get Healthy

In this chapter, we introduced a number of the tools, tactics, and information you need to start getting healthy. Hang tight, because in Chapter 4, we'll help you make sense of all of the information, to build it into a practical protocol that doesn't break the bank.

But before then, I need to come back to this concept of slowing down to get healthy. I won't name names, but you may have read chapters like this, and your mind is probably racing in anticipation of solving problems and belly-flopping into the deep end. Not to be a broken record, but you can't heal in a state of stress. Take some deep breaths. If you're going to introduce anything to your life at this point, let it be the ability to de-stress.

If something crazy happened to you, and your stress level was a 10 out of 10, what would you do to bring it down to a 5 out of 10? What I've found is that most people have an answer. One of my patients told me she'd go out on her own to just sit by the river. I love that! But here's the convicting part: When I asked her when the last time was that she did just that, she couldn't think of an answer. Does that describe you? You might have a clear picture in your mind of what you'd do to settle yourself, but you aren't putting it into action!

Ask yourself this: What do you even do for fun? A coach asked me this question, and I have to admit that it took me a moment to even come up with the answer. It had me pulling out a guitar for the first time in a very long time, just so I could reintroduce the habit into my life.

Are you able to slow down? To make healthy nutrition decisions, practice breathwork, and incorporate manageable movement? If I can convince you of one thing in this book, I hope it's that perimenopause isn't as simple as introducing the right hormone therapies. On the contrary, I want to be the first person to tell you that they won't work as they should unless you address the stressed out, rushed, possibly damaging lifestyle that you might be living.

3.
SYMPTOMS, LAB TESTS, AND THE PURSUIT OF THE IDEAL DAY

This is a chapter about symptoms and making sense of them—the last step before building a protocol. But before we go there, we have to take a detour to somewhere much more pleasant: your ideal day. Think about this, a successful journey that has a destination in mind. Many women have vague ideas of what it looks like to experience healing and living without being at the mercy of their symptoms, but few have more than that.

I'm a big believer in something called the Ideal Day exercise. In this exercise, you take pen to paper and, in vivid detail, you describe the perfect day. Here's the crazy part: Your brain can't distinguish between reality and something richly imagined. If you do this properly, you should be able to place yourself in the shoes of a happier, healthier you. To what end? Well, the goal is to motivate you to move toward this beacon of light at the end of the tunnel.

With a goal in mind, you're empowered to go farther. If you followed along, you already completed the State of the Union exercise (page 24). That's the dose of reality. The Ideal Day exercise isn't limited by what you currently think is possible. In mine, I was bold enough to place myself and my family in Hawaii. So, in the writing exercise, that's where I woke up. I made coffee, ate delicious food, and experienced warm embraces. I felt exercise replenishing my body and the sun kissing my skin. I went on a date with my girl—I was in paradise.

In writing, you shouldn't be cold and distant. You should activate all five senses—what do you taste, touch, smell, see, and hear? If you can't put yourselves in the shoes of yourself in this exercise, you're doing it wrong. One of my patients went through this exercise and wrote out seven pages of information. When she read it back to me and I closed my eyes, it was as if I were in a movie. She was exploring specific shops in Banff, eating a dinner with grandchildren, enjoying a dish she specifically described, and had a specific hobby project she was working on.

What about you? It might sound woo-woo, but if you want to bring the pinprick of light at the end of the tunnel closer, your brain has to be able to at least imagine the possibility of it in detail.

This isn't an exercise about moving to paradise, but in my example, it actually played out in my life. We did move to Hawaii for a period of time. I guess you could say to be careful what you chase after, because you might just catch it.

A Pipe Dream Is Your Secret Weapon

When I describe this exercise, so many of the women I speak to have the same question: Why does that matter? Why would I just depress myself further by imagining something so unachievable? Actually, the woman I was describing, who wrote seven pages for this exercise, felt that way. She had multiple autoimmune diseases, she was in the midst of menopause, and there was a lot to unpack in her life.

I get it. Imagining something so idealistic feels intellectually dishonest to our present circumstances, sometimes. But that's why we did the State of the Union exercise (page 24). That exercise holds space for the reality of the present situation. But on the other hand, so many women end up so far inside the box they can't even read the label. Many times, we put ourselves in these boxes without even retaining the capability to understand how we ended up there in the first place.

By the way, the State of the Union exercise shouldn't just capture symptoms. It should capture the state of the relationships you have in your life, your overall satisfaction with the life you've built, and everything else you can think of that would encapsulate your present state. If you were to dump everything out onto a friend or therapist, what would you say? Write it down here.

At the end of the day, if you know where you are and have an idea of where you want to go, you can look back every couple of months and gauge where you are on your journey. A distinct Point A–to–Point B journey can go a long way, compared to random wandering down unknown paths. What people ultimately realize once they've done this is that, when it comes time for a check-in, they might not be at their destination yet, but they can identify that they aren't at the place they began.

The Hormone Cascade Starts with What?

We're about to dive into an ultra-practical symptoms checklist that will help you identify where you stand in regard to hormone-related symptoms. Before we do, I want to remind you, very briefly, of the hormone cascade. In the body, all of these hormones are being converted from different forms into their bioavailable states.

If you recall, every hormone starts with cholesterol. It then goes to pregnenolone. Pregnenolone then shifts into a progesterone side and an androgen side. On the androgen side is DHEA, which then converts into testosterone. Through something called aromatase, testosterone can then be converted into estrogen. There are many forms of estrogen, but estradiol (E2) is the most prevalent.

Think of this as a stream where one river turns into many smaller branches. We start with cholesterol, but then we trickle downstream into the hormones progesterone, testosterone, and estrogen, among others. You don't need to have this memorized, but it can help to understand—especially as shifts in cholesterol come into the conversation as part of perimenopause!

The Ultimate Perimenopause Symptoms Checklist

Western medicine has led us all to believe in one cause, one cure. I've received hundreds of messages from men and women that essentially boil down to prodding about which one supplement or prescription they need. This desperate digging for a silver bullet is perpetuated by videos online, doctors, and others who overpromise and underdeliver.

The reality is, this approach undersells the complexity of the human body. We're not looking for one singular cause. We're looking for multiple causes, and we're equipping the body to take on the stressors, deficiencies, and imbalances.

Let's take a run back through the key hormones in the perimenopause conversation. But this time, let's focus on the symptoms. See how many boxes you're checking in each category. Understand that checking the boxes alone isn't a medical diagnosis. And yet, the clues can be helpful as we work together to build a protocol in the next chapter.

Symptoms Caused by Estrogen

Remember: Rarely, if ever, is estrogen deficiency an issue in perimenopause. In perimenopause, most women are producing more estrogen than ever before . . . in their entire life! I can't be clear enough in saying estrogen deficiency is rare. Now, estrogen *dominance* is possible. However, in many cases, estrogen dominance is really a progesterone deficiency. And as a review, progesterone deficiency is, I would argue, the consensus in research as the most common deficiency in perimenopause.

I also want to acknowledge that if you're reading this and you're in menopause rather than perimenopause, it is true that you will have practically no estrogen in your system. What happens is that the ovaries make one last, huge push during the years of perimenopause, and finally surrender during menopause. To be clear, menopause is defined by the time that you have not had any menstrual cycle for 12 months consecutively.

Alright, let's dive into the estrogen symptoms. We'll start by reviewing the symptoms of a deficiency, and then we'll look at the symptoms of having excessive estrogen. If you're checking a lot of boxes in the deficiency category, I also want you to be mindful later on for other hormones that may be implicated for those same symptoms. Just to make things confusing, there's a lot of overlap among the different hormones' causing similar symptoms.

Estrogen Deficiency Symptoms

- Hot flashes
- Night sweats
- Depression
- Brain fog
- Fatigue/low energy
- Weight gain
- Vaginal dryness
- Urinary tract infections
- Decreased libido
- Pain during intercourse
- Urinary leakage
- Droopy breast tissue
- Dry, dehydrated skin
- Thinning skin
- Loss of glow
- Dry eyes
- Vertical lines around mouth
- High cholesterol (in any form)
- Back and joint pain
- Low bone density

Excessive Estrogen Symptoms

- Breast tenderness
- Breast fullness
- Nipple tenderness
- Fluid retention

Symptoms Caused by Progesterone

Remember, when we discuss progesterone, that what should come to mind is a brake pedal. Slowing down, deep breaths. In the menstrual cycle, it's natural for specific phases to be progesterone dominant and for it to sink back down during other phases. But what we're looking for here are symptoms of an across-the-board progesterone deficiency.

Progesterone Deficiency Symptoms

- Difficulty falling asleep and staying asleep
- Irritability/short fuse
- Mood swings
- Swollen, painful breast tissue
- Fibrocystic breast tissue
- Swollen feet and ankles
- Period irregularities (shortened period)
- Scanty menstrual flow
- Heavy menstrual flow
- Premenstrual syndrome (PMS)
- Endometriosis or fibroids
- History of infertility
- History of miscarriage
- Headaches
- Acne
- Swollen face
- Low bone density
- Anxiety
- Inability to relax
- Hot flashes

Progesterone Excess Symptoms

I don't have a checklist for you in this category, but one is telltale—drowsiness. If you find yourself unable to even stay awake throughout the day, you might just have a progesterone excess problem rather than a deficiency.

Symptoms Caused by Testosterone

For a moment, think back to the hormone cascade we introduced near the beginning of this chapter. We're on the androgen side of the hormone cascade. Testosterone is ultimately converted from DHEA, so as we consider the symptoms caused by testosterone imbalance, we can have DHEA in mind as well.

Testosterone is a necessary part of a woman's hormonal balance, though it's often villainized or even feared. Most women don't want to come anywhere near to having high testosterone. And, yes, the symptoms of high testosterone in women can be unpleasant. But what's not talked about much is how difficult the symptoms of low testosterone can be.

As with all the hormones, the goal is not to be high or low. The goal is to find healthy balance. Don't neglect testosterone!

Testosterone Deficiency Symptoms

- Loss of muscle
- Abdominal weight gain
- Cellulite
- Varicose veins
- Loss of libido
- Lack of orgasm

- Low clitoral sensitivity
- Dry eyes
- Loss of confidence
- Low energy and stamina
- Immune dysfunction
- Digestive issues
- Poor tissue repair
- Low bone density

Excessive Testosterone Symptoms
- Unwanted hair growth (excessive)
- Voice changes and deepening
- Aggression
- Oily skin
- Loss of hair on the head
- Acne

Symptoms Caused by the Thyroid

Thyroid hormones play an instrumental role in perimenopause. Many women are aware that they have imbalances here, whereas others have suffered unknowingly. By the way, another reminder is warranted that just because your doctor says you're normal in your lab results does not mean you can skip this section. First of all, did your doctor even run a full thyroid panel, or just a couple of markers? If you do have the full panel, are you normal only in the sense of being in range? We're not just looking for that; we're looking for *optimal*.

Underactive Thyroid Symptoms

- Fatigue/low energy
- Weight gain
- Difficulty losing weight
- Cold sensitivity
- Cold hands or feet
- Dry skin
- Dry hair
- Constipation
- Depression or low mood
- Muscle cramps and weakness
- Slowed heart rate
- Puffy face and swelling
- Irregular or heavy periods
- Elevated cholesterol levels
- Thinning of the lateral third of the eyebrow
- Brittle nails

Overactive Thyroid Symptoms

- Uncontrollable weight loss
- Anxiety
- Heat sensitivity
- Rapid heart rate
- Increased hunger
- Tremors
- Brittle hair
- Irregular periods

Symptoms Caused by Insulin

Back to the insulin conversation. Insulin, of course, is made most famous by its associations with blood sugar and diabetes. A term that's coming into the limelight is insulin resistance. Many, many people experience insulin resistance at some level, and you could be one of them. Remember, insulin resistance is most often determined by high levels of insulin on a fasting insulin lab test. This is because the body is producing insulin, but the cells are not allowing the utilization of it. Let's dive into the checklist and see whether it resonates.

Insulin Resistance Symptoms
- Trembling
- Sweating
- Dizziness
- Lightheadedness
- Hunger/feeling hangry
- Fatigue
- Headaches
- Blurred vision
- Irritability
- Mood swings

Symptoms Caused by Melatonin

Remember, we're not talking about the sleep aid supplements! It's true that melatonin does most of its work during the night and around sleep. But when we address it here, we're talking about the hormone naturally produced by your body. Many people will find that they have issues with melatonin, which can explain restlessness, among many other symptoms.

Low Melatonin Symptoms

- Insomnia
- Difficulty falling asleep
- Frequently waking
- Poor-quality sleep
- Daytime fatigue
- Mood disturbances
- Decreased cognitive function
- Increased sensitivity to light
- Weakened immune function

Symptoms Caused by Vitamin D

Vitamin D is the hormone that most people have never called a hormone. This is easily one of the most deficient hormones I see across the many, many lab tests I've helped people run. You'll see fatigue again on this list, but I want to make special note of it. More so than almost anything else, optimizing vitamin D levels is among the most impactful ways to fight fatigue for the average person. Our clients constantly report higher energy levels as a result of raising their vitamin D levels.

Low Vitamin D Symptoms

- Fatigue
- Bone pain
- Muscle weakness
- Low mood/depression
- Increased risk of infection
- Hair loss

Tying the Hormones Symptoms Back Together

If you're thinking, "Wow, they're all intertwined!" you're exactly right. It begs the question, "Where do you start?" This is an important part of the conversation. I've said it before and I'll say it again—you should never add more than one thing at a time. If you did, how would we know what works for you? Or if something's not working, how would we know that? The only way is to introduce things one by one.

I get it. You want to start five things so you can feel better than ever . . . tomorrow! But here's the problem: Let's assume something didn't work. Let's assume none of it worked! How can we possibly know why? It could be that the different things you're taking interacted with one another in ways that made them ineffective. It could be that, sure enough, none or only some of these options were the missing ingredients for you. But we'd never know, because there were too many variables introduced all at once.

On the other hand, if it does work, we have no idea why. Now you're stuck taking all five of those things, at the risk of peeling one back and returning to your prior state. Twenty years of being a doctor has taught me to have good conversations with people. To dive into symptomatology. To find the first domino in the line!

If you're looking at your sheet of checkmarks and finding that they're all full, take a deep breath. We'll find the starting place, and we'll move forward one step at a time. And by the way, don't forget that we're talking energy and drainage, before we're even beginning to talk about optimizing hormones.

Signals, Not Symptoms

When we can take three steps back and understand neurology, pathophysiology, and cellular biochemistry (along with some other really big, long words), we learn that the body responds appropriately to its environment. I want to be clear—I'm not pro-symptom. I don't cheer for symptoms and I understand how debilitating, frustrating, uncomfortable, and painful they can be.

But in one sense, I want to have appreciation for what we can learn from a symptom. A symptom is really more like a signal—it's the "check engine" light in your car. A symptom gives us clues about what actually matters—the cause.

Women come into my practice all the time with statements like this one: "My symptoms all started five years ago." Interesting! If you're someone who can pinpoint something like this, I'm glad you have the self-awareness to be able to understand the before vs the after. Most people probably don't realize how interesting I find these statements. But my follow-up to that question is this: "What was going on in your life five years ago?"

What if we assume that your body is profoundly intelligent? (By the way, there's a good case for that.) The more you learn about how intricate your body is, the more you can appreciate how intelligent its responses are. You can understand how trillions of cells, millions of bits of information being passed around each second, and highly intricate processes, such as even maintaining pH balance, suggest that your body is adept at responding to a wide variety of situations and circumstances.

Sometimes, we get frustrated by our symptoms. Fatigue is frustrating; unchecked weight gain makes us want to pull our hair out ... but what if we paused first? What if we considered why our body is throwing a symptom at us in the first place? What could it be responding to?

Let's come back to my patient who said this had all started five years ago. We went back in time together. I guided her through a series of questions, and it came to light that she had been handling a high-stress corporate job and a divorce. Remember that the body can't distinguish forms of stress, so these mental and emotional stressors can have the same impact in triggering disease processes as any other form of stress.

But that's not all. She also brought up that she had been in the middle of a bathroom renovation at that time. When they gutted the bathroom, they found out it was covered in mold. Interesting. That's an environmental stressor and certain molds are powerful toxins. When all of the elements come together, the way they did for her, we call that the perfect storm. The only problem is that neither you nor your doctor are trained to consider these elements when you look into your symptoms.

Here's an example. If I were to walk out of the room I'm sitting in right now and trip on something, I'd bring it up to my doctor. In fact, I'd go as far as to say it would be crazy if I didn't. Can you imagine going to your doctor in pain from this circumstance and neither of you considered the cause? In acute cases, it's super easy to correlate cause and effect.

But what's harder to pinpoint are micro-events that stack up over time, causing chronic symptoms to rear their ugly heads. Let's say you have a bacterial overgrowth—your body will come to bat to fight against this. But then, let's layer in emotional stress—a kid who's not doing well, or a stressful relationship. At this point, your body's plate is full.

Worse yet? Something inconspicuous. Maybe you're exposed to a virus or something. This small thing should have been easily handled by your body. But the problem is the plate was already full, and now it's spilling over. It stumps us every time. We fail to put all of the pieces together and tell the story, instead going about our lives as usual when, suddenly, the wheels fall off for no apparent reason. What you didn't see was the plate slowly filling up. When you catch only the last event that caused the spill, nothing else that actually preceded it adds up.

Let symptoms drive curiosity. Let your body tell you that something is up. Going back to the "check engine" lights example, good mechanics don't just scratch their head and walk away; they search the code and discover the cause for the light's turning on in the first place. And by the way, they don't just try to turn off the light; they look for the root cause.

Once they know the cause, some people might bring up the fact that the car was driving fine up until that moment. You and your mechanics should be grateful that the light came on instead of the motor exploding. You and they should both be grateful at this point that you didn't just put a piece of black electrical tape over the light to make it less annoying.

Lab Work for Perimenopause

If you've ever seen one of my videos on social media or heard me speak, you're probably well aware that I am a big fan of lab testing. And not just lab testing—comprehensive lab testing. So, hopefully, it means something to hear this from me, but in the case of perimenopause, symptoms trump lab test values. Especially when you start to get into the art of hormones.

Speaking of the art and the science, the science of lab test values is what I love. Laboratories have gotten good at lab testing and there's a high level of precision in the results you get back. This isn't about doubting the numbers on the paper. But the art of medicine, and especially hormones, comes into play when we look at those values. We know where a person ideally should be from a numbers perspective, but what we've learned is that doesn't always mean that person feels optimal, even when the numbers suggest it.

One difficult thing about hormone testing should be noted here. Unlike many lab tests, those for hormones' optimal level are not universal. What we find is that "optimal" looks different for everyone. The best ways to find your optimal level are by correlating your results with your symptoms and by taking a much larger data set into consideration. Consider all the other lab tests you may have had at around this time. Many of those markers have more definitive optimal ranges. If they are in balance, your hormones are within reference ranges, and you have few symptoms, you can consider that optimal.

Sex Hormone Lab Tests

Before we go too deep into the weeds, let's start introducing some of the tests that can be run. We'll start with the sex hormones. By running these tests, you might get some definitive proof to back the assumptions you just made when completing The Ultimate Perimenopause Symptoms Checklist (page 87). Remember that high *or* low levels of each sex hormone have a whole list of symptoms they can trigger.

You might also recall that tricky element of the checklist: how the same symptom can have several potential causes that are vastly different from one another. Sex hormone lab tests can help clear up that confusion—don't discard the symptoms checklist. Instead, use it to correlate your test findings with how you really feel.

Finally, understand that sex hormones vary tremendously, depending on where you are at in your menstrual cycle. Most labs or physicians should tell you when they would like you to test in the cycle. The reference ranges in the test should correlate with that point in your cycle. There are times in your cycle where certain hormones surge and others diminish. Most of the insight isn't from the number you get as a result—it's from correlating that result with the other hormones to understand the ratios between them.

- Estradiol
- Progesterone
- Free testosterone
- Total testosterone
- DHEA (DHEA-S)

Thyroid Lab Tests

Right off the bat, I want to tell you that my very favorite lab test for the thyroid measures free T3. Free T3 is an unbound, bioavailable thyroid hormone. It has a tremendous impact on your metabolism, among many other key functions. So, if you're having thyroid lab tests, you need to get your free T3 number. However, you also want to know free T4. It's good to know your TSH, and it's really good to know reverse T3. That leads us to whether there are antithyroid antibodies—at this point, we've arrived at the full thyroid panel.

For free T3, there is an optimal result I want you to keep in mind. We're aiming for 3.0+. Even if a lab test's reference range says you're "in range," check to see whether you're above 3.0. If not, I would consider you to be below optimal in this area. And if that's the case, follow Chapter 4's discussion of thyroid protocols closely.

Let's break it down:
- Free T3 (optimal: 3.0 or higher)
- Free T4
- TSH
- Reverse T3
- Anti-TPO
- Anti-TG

Metabolic Lab Tests

When it comes to metabolic lab tests, I like to test specifically for *fasting* insulin and fasting glucose. The goal of the fasting insulin test is to understand whether you have proper insulin sensitivity or you've become insulin resistant. This is a key piece of the puzzle. The fasting insulin number is another key result to track. This time, you're aiming for the optimal range of 2 to 8. If you're higher than that, I'd consider you to be insulin resistant or on the road to it.

- Fasting insulin (optimal: 2–8)
- Hemoglobin A1C
- Fasting glucose

Adrenal Lab Tests

Lots of people have different opinions on the ideal way to do adrenal lab testing. My preference is salivary testing, which helps us map out your day—we've talked about things like the cortisol waking response, and a multipoint salivary test can help us track these responses throughout your day.

Vitamin D Lab Test

One of the simplest lab tests that you can take is for vitamin D. Don't overcomplicate this one! Remember that vitamin D is a hormone, and it's another key result. The aim is to fall within the range of 60 to 80 here.

- 25-hydroxy vitamin D (optimal: 60–80)

Inflammatory Lab Test

I like looking at inflammatory markers, for a number of reasons. It's been said that inflammation plays a role in every single disease process that can be experienced by the body. We can do all kinds of other work to support your body, but if every cell inside you is practically on fire, it won't help! Knowing where inflammatory markers stand helps us get a good piece of the overall picture.

High-sensitivity C-reactive protein (HS-CRP) is a key result in such tests. Typically, a lab's reference range for this will consider up to 1.0 to be "in range" but I prefer you to be less than 0.3. Even low-level inflammation can wreak havoc in the body.

- HS-CRP (optimal: 0.3 or less)

Anemia Lab Test

Do you know whether you're anemic? If not, this is an important piece of understanding to have.

- Ferritin
- Iron
- Hematocrit

Methylation Lab Test

You've probably heard a bit about liver detoxes. The liver actually detoxifies itself regularly. Its process for doing so has two key phases. In the second phase, a biochemical process called methylation comes into play. Methylation is beneficial for the body in numerous ways. Unfortunately, some people don't methylate well, which creates issues.

One key reason to understand whether you're methylating effectively is the impact the process has on clearing estrogen. If you're not methylating well, you might be storing up harmful estrogen metabolites in your body, contributing to hormone issues of all kinds.

- Homocysteine

Drainage Lab Test

If your drainage system isn't doing its job, we're not going to make a lot of progress. Some of these lab tests can help you get a grasp on what's going on. We'll focus on tests that give us a peek at some of the essential drainage organs: the kidneys, liver, and gut. By the way, this involves a lot of markers. Thankfully, they are available in a very common panel called the comprehensive metabolic profile (CMP).

- Liver: enzyme panel (albumin, AST, ALT, alkaline phosphatase, bilirubin)
- Kidneys: sodium, creatinine, estimated glomerular filtration rate (eGFR), blood urea nitrogen (BUN)
- Gut: total protein, BUN

Why These Lab Tests?

In your mind, the idea of running a bunch of lab tests that aren't specifically hormone panels might seem questionable. To the contrary, the nonhormone lab tests I have listed here are the most important. The reason we can't truly look at hormone lab tests and find "optimal" is that there are 10 ways hormone receptivity can be hijacked within the body. And if this happens, you have absolutely no chance of your body *using* the available hormones optimally even if their *levels* are optimal.

By the way, there are additional tests that could offer valuable insight if you have had a tougher case. Maybe you've already had some of them and aren't getting answers. Maybe you're taking stout doses of hormones and not seeing results. In this case, you might consider a specific lab panel that measures the presence of endocrine-disrupting chemicals in the body. High levels could be one of the ways your hormones are ultimately hijacked.

The lab tests listed in this chapter help provide a picture of how your body is actually utilizing your hormones and what stands in the way of better efficiency. So, yes, if all of your other lab results are optimal, you can actually feel optimal. And that's the ultimate goal, right?

Learn to identify what "optimal" feels like to you! For instance, having optimal progesterone feels like a sense of ease. The ability to rest and relax. Optimal DHEA and testosterone offer a feeling of resilience. You'll feel that you have some "get up and go." If you know you don't feel optimal, but don't know why, refer back to your Ultimate Perimenopause Symptoms Checklist (page 87). Take note of overlapping symptoms that may have multiple causes, but look intently for where patterns emerge. Which category has the greatest number of checkmarks?

For an extra assurance, consider running through the checklist once for each week of your menstrual cycle, to see whether anything changes. If you did run labs, you can also identify how the symptoms and the lab results are correlated.

Are You Hormone Resistant?

I just alluded to 10 ways that hormone receptivity can be hijacked. We don't need to go through all of them, but I do want you to know that it's important to grasp whether your body is resistant to hormones. We've made sense of this phenomenon with something many are familiar with—insulin resistance. In this circumstance, we find insulin in the body, but identify that it's not able to be received by the cells.

What's interesting is we don't talk as much about the very real existence of progesterone resistance, testosterone resistance, and estradiol resistance. If you're that person who's been taking mammoth doses of hormones without moving the needle, you might be someone who is experiencing hormone resistance.

Oh, and by the way, have you seen your hormone test results improve into optimal levels, but don't feel any different? This is probably a case of hormone resistance, too!

Resistance brings us back to my example of dumping gasoline all over a car. Gas makes cars go, but it doesn't help unless it's loaded into the gas tank.

We also run lab tests to ensure that there isn't any pathology standing in the way of your feeling like yourself. Many times, women don't even realize they've been carrying chronic issues for years or decades. If they are, identifying and addressing such issues become part of the journey as well.

At the end of the day, this is where the State of the Union exercise (page 24) comes back into play. I recommend doing it every time you go in for lab testing. The goal is to associate the numbers on paper with how they actually make you feel. That way, we don't lose track of you and start jockeying numbers—we address how you're feeling and associate that with the numbers.

When to Have Lab Testing

For women, it's essential to consider their menstrual cycle before scheduling lab testing. Keep in mind it's totally normal and healthy for hormones to fluctuate throughout the cycle. That needs to be accounted for. Most bioidentical hormone experts have a preference for specific days of the cycle—oftentimes, within the luteal phase (just after ovulation). By the way, if you're among those women who experience irregular cycles and don't even reach such days? That's okay, too; just communicate with your practitioner or whoever it is that's ordering the lab testing for you.

Even if you're ordering your own lab tests at home, it might still be worthwhile to ensure that you have a chance to communicate with an expert in at least a brief consultation, to ensure that you understand these numbers, especially in light of your cycle.

If at all possible, it is preferable to do lab testing before starting a treatment protocol. This allows you to get a true baseline for where you stand before taking any action. If you've already started or have been taking steps for your health for some time, you should at least pause any supplementation for five days prior to running lab tests, if it is safe to do so.

A Note about Optimal Numbers for Lab Results

We've already laid out the disclaimer that not every woman whose lab testing results are "optimal" feels optimal. And yet, there's value in understanding some of these ranges for the key lab test values. We already mentioned that the sex hormones have no true ideal range, so that leaves us with the remaining hormones on our list of important players in perimenopause: thyroid hormones, insulin, vitamin D, and melatonin. In the case of melatonin, you're best off determining what is "optimal" by the quality and quantity of the sleep you're able to get. For the remaining hormones, your practitioner can provide optimal ranges.

If you're whipping out lab testing results you've already run, remember that the ranges you'll see in this book are smaller than those you see on the lab report in your hand. Laboratory reference ranges are based on averages from sample groups. Falling outside those ranges can indicate that you're way off base from "normal" and could even be in a diagnosable disease state or dealing with a deficiency, depending on the marker. My ranges are smaller. If you fall outside them, you might appear normal in lab results while feeling nothing like it. That's because you're outside what I would consider the optimal range.

Correlating Labs

The real art of running lab tests is correlating all of these separate markers. We have to understand how the liver and the kidneys link back to drainage and how that impacts the hormones. We have to know what kind of impact rampant inflammation or poor methylation have on the body.

On top of that, can we understand the state of your nervous system, to know whether you're capable of resting, digesting, and healing? Oh, and of course, if you have very little progesterone, you might have some of the same symptoms as a nervous system in the fight-or-flight state. Yikes—there's a lot to take in here.

My aim isn't to make things sound confusing. There are so many factors involved. For instance, age, proximity to menopause, and other key factors can shift what we'd hope to be optimal for such things like DHEA and estradiol. Symptoms trump lab tests. Yes, I'm a huge advocate for lab testing, and I encourage you to get the most comprehensive set of lab tests that's feasibly possible. And yet? Symptoms trump lab tests.

A Note on Ordering Lab Tests

Depending on the laws in your locale, most of us now enjoy more flexibility than ever when ordering lab work. The benefit of working with your practitioner is that you (hopefully) get their expert analysis along with the values in the lab test results themselves. The downside is that many practitioners become obstinate about ordering lab tests they don't typically run, and of course, most of them don't share the same viewpoint on what those numbers mean. Many times, patients will get no more analysis than a quick "looks good."

But these days, you have other options—you can actually order virtually any lab test yourself, in most areas. Some can be taken at home, some can be ordered and sent to a local phlebotomist. Use the URL in the Resources section of this book to take you to a compilation of my lab testing recommendations, so that they're easy to identify and order. Alternatively, you can find a variety of options online for purchasing them yourself.

A Framework for Perimenopause

In these first three chapters, we've put together the framework for an approach to perimenopause that gets the results many women are looking for. There's no "Easy" button, and skipping steps doesn't pay off, but patience and following these steps does see results. It begins with cellular energy and the understanding that nothing "goes" without gas in the tank. We move to drainage. Your body's always dumping things into a drainage funnel, and if they don't come out efficiently enough, you get overflow. Sometimes, it looks like skin reactions; sometimes, it's constipation or an inability to sweat (among many other symptoms).

From drainage, we go into optimizing hormones and clearing interference. The effects of interference range from endocrine-disrupting chemicals to stress of all kinds, toxins, infections, and more. And of course, at the base of it all, we work on nervous system regulation, with the understanding that fight-or-flight responses inhibit healing.

I get it. That's a lot of steps. That's not a *take this for that* approach. But I get hundreds of messages on social media from women who tried a *this for that* approach and found it to be a failure. So, that's why we take the extra steps to do this right. In the next chapter, we'll unpack the protocol in more detail, so that you can build one that works.

4.
TAKING ON PERIMENOPAUSE: BUILD YOUR PROTOCOL

We've spent half of this book laying a foundation, and now it's time to put the knowledge into practice. We're going to work together to build a perimenopause protocol. Now, I do need to offer a caveat, something that's probably no surprise—as I can't possibly grasp the unique circumstances each of my readers experiences as they read this chapter, I can't build a protocol for you without having a personal relationship with you. Ultimately, you may need to have a relationship with a physician or expert who directly oversees what you're doing. That said, you will be able to maintain a regular relationship with your primary-care doctor while taking on the day-to-day of this on your own. It depends which route you choose to.

Now, what I *can* help you do is make sense of all of the individual building blocks that I've set out in front of us. I can help you construct a foundation, and I can give you some blueprints based on paths women like you have walked. I'm here to come alongside you for each step.

This chapter will be ultra-tactical. By the end of it, my goal is for you to have constructed the first draft of your own protocol. In Chapter 5, we'll learn about making responsible tweaks to that protocol. We'll also dive into how to approach something that isn't working without panicking or thinking that you have lost all reason for hope.

Hopefully, if you've learned one thing from this book, it's to pause before running to a hormone clinic. We've explored the significance of energy, drainage, and the state of your nervous system. We've introduced the concepts of hormone resistance as well. Now, it's time to put the pieces in play.

Step One: Correlating Symptoms with Lab Testing

In the previous chapter, I laid out a bunch of lab tests that should be on the radar of women in perimenopause. I also emphasized why, at the end of the day, symptoms trump labs. Hopefully, I've hit that point hard enough that you've already taken the time to fill out the Ultimate Perimenopause Symptoms Checklist (page 87). I would also hope that you've completed the State of the Union exercise (page 24). If you haven't, now's your chance. By the way, circle back to the State of the Union and the symptoms checklist every few months. You'd be amazed how many women don't realize that they've made any progress, until they look back at where they've come from.

As we mentioned before, the best time to do lab testing is before beginning a treatment protocol. You might be in a position to run all of those that I recommended. Otherwise, you may need to pick and choose. I also want to introduce you to a specific hormone test that I believe can be beneficial. This panel is called the Hormone Zoomer. As I've stated previously, hormone markers really don't have optimal ranges. However, this test can help us understand how your body is clearing estrogen.

Remember that estrogen is typically dominant in perimenopause. If it can't be cleared out of the body effectively, estrogen dominance becomes a major possibility. Keep in mind that a lot of this work is done by your liver, and that's a huge part of the reason that I recommended the liver enzyme panel as a key lab test in the last chapter. However, the Hormone Zoomer is an interesting panel, as it also gives you a snapshot of any presence of endocrine-disrupting chemicals in your body.

If you recall, endocrine-disrupting chemicals are the ones that can mimic real hormones in your body, ultimately damaging hormone receptivity. If we can understand how high the levels of these chemicals are in your body, it paints part of the picture. We can start to understand why hormone imbalances, deficiencies, or excess become possible. Bisphenol A (BPA), just one of the many endocrine-disrupting chemicals, can itself inhibit hormone receptivity in 6 of the 10 different ways possible to do so.

So, if you're going to run a hormone test, the Hormone Zoomer panel is my recommendation. But to go back to all of the other testing I recommended in the previous chapter, there were an almost overwhelming number of markers to measure. The good news is that many come grouped together in lab panels. You don't have to order each of these tests one by one. Look for the comprehensive metabolic profile (CMP), a full thyroid panel, and, again, the Hormone Zoomer. If you start with those three panels, you'll have covered many of the bases. You'll only have to worry about a couple of additional markers, such as for vitamin D, which typically are ordered separately.

Step Two: Build a Drainage & Energy Protocol

We went over a hefty amount of information on drainage and cellular energy in Chapter 1. I won't rehash it here, so make sure to go back to the beginning of this book, to dive back into the information surrounding this. Essentially, the important thing is to make sure your drainage pathways are wide open and your cellular energy is sufficient.

We listed a lot of tactics in Chapter 1, but how does that look in a protocol? The first thing I want you to know about this phase is that it's not a "one and done." Drainage and cellular energy are always a component in your protocol. So, when we consider that protocol, we have to be mindful of building something sustainable that can be maintained.

Here's how to build that protocol from square one. Remember, it's okay to ease things in. The more you slow down, the more aware you become of what's actually working. You might find yourself getting overwhelmed trying to figure all of this out, and that's exactly the time to slow down.

Increase Your Water Intake: No excuses—start drinking more water. As much as you don't want to think so, you're probably dehydrated. Ideally, you'd drink at least half your body weight in fluid ounces every day. So, if you're 180 pounds (82 kg), you'd want to drink 90 fluid ounces (2.7 L) of water throughout the day. That's just over 11 cups (2.6 L) of water. If you can, filter the water to reduce toxins carried by it. Increase your intake slowly to build up to your daily goal, and focus on sustaining this habit.

Based on Your Lab Results, Look at Liver Support: If, as for many women, your liver is struggling, there's one last supplement that is well worth considering. Tauroursodeoxycholic acid (TUDCA) is an ingredient that has changed the game for many women. There are no miracle pills, but TUDCA packs a serious punch when it comes to liver support. This can be a costly supplement, especially if it comes from a good source, but for some women, this is a must.

Increase Your Protein & Fatty Acid Intake: Ensure protein is meaningfully included in every meal. In the morning, incorporate Greek yogurt, eggs, or meat. For lunch and dinner, high-quality cheeses and meats should be on your plate. A huge portion of women suffer hidden consequences from rampant protein deficiency. Finally, get in fatty acids, too. Ditch your vegetable oil and opt for olive oil or beef tallow.

Grab a Mitochondrial Support Supplement: Supplements are ever improving. In the Resources (page 185), follow the URL to my best recommendations, and revisit the site periodically so you can keep them up to date. I won't recommend a specific product here since the best options change, but the supplement you're ultimately looking for will be an antioxidant powerhouse with such ingredients as NAC, ALA, ALC, and resveratrol. It should also incorporate micronutrients that help feed your cells.

Get in a 20-Minute Walk . . . Daily: You can move your body however you'd like, but the easiest way to incorporate movement is a brisk 20-minute walk every day. This supports both energy and drainage.

Hack Your Sleep: Review the list of sleep recommendations in Chapter 1. Most of these ask very little of you, so maybe you can incorporate them all. Try at least a couple, to see whether you can improve the quantity and quality of your sleep. If you're not sleeping optimally, you're not healing optimally.

Cut Out Toxins: Stop using antiperspirant and purge your house of the toxins you consume or utilize most frequently.

Consider an As-Needed Drainage Supplement: Yes, this is another supplement, the third I've recommended so far. The good news is that a drainage supplement doesn't need to be taken every day. Buy a high-quality supplement and use it for extra support only when you're backed up. If you're not having daily bowel movements, it might be a good time to slip this in.

By the way, other great options for the liver include potent antioxidants, such as glutathione or silymarin (from milk thistle).

Rotate Drainage Tactics: In Chapter 1, we shared a number of tools and tactics for supporting drainage. We broke it down by system. So, if you have had lab testing and know what's up, select tactics from the list that offer targeted support to that system. If you don't know which to try, pick a few tactics that seem to fit best with your lifestyle. The goal is to get into the habit of supporting drainage and have a sense for what works.

To summarize, here's your energy and drainage protocol:
- Drink half of your body weight in pounds (1 lb = .45 kg) in fluid ounces of water (1 oz = 30 ml) gradually throughout the day.
- Consume 1 to 1.5 grams of protein per pound (.45 kg) of body weight.
- Switch to olive oil or beef tallow for cooking.
- Grab a mitochondrial support supplement.
- Find time for 20-minute daily walks.
- Hack your sleep.
- Reduce your toxic load by cutting out household toxins.
- Rotate your drainage support tactics.
- Consider nonlaxative support for constipation (as needed).
- Consider liver support supplementation (as needed).

What's your reaction to that? Does that sound completely doable, or does it look like a nightmare? Take note of your reaction and ask yourself—would it be worth it to get well? Hopefully, the answer's yes. At the end of the day, this entire list boils down to a few things: Make some healthy swaps, drink more water, move more, sleep well, and offer extra support with supplements and drainage tactics.

Start slow, but don't deprioritize. If you skip to the hormones, you can't be surprised when things don't work out well.

Step Three: Maintain the State of Your Nervous System

It's fairly easy to self-assess the state of your nervous system if you have the ability to be honest with yourself. Go back to our previous conversations about this, if you need more information. But as we've discussed, your nervous system can actually prevent healing if it's perpetually in a fight-or-flight state. Dealing with insane amounts of stress to your system (in any form) is bound to leave you frustrated and not making any progress.

For some women, nervous system work is on an as-needed basis. Others may be so frazzled and frustrated that they need to focus time and energy on this daily. The good news is that this work should be the best part of your day. You should feel rested, recovered, and at ease when you're done. I do want you to remember the fact that progesterone deficiency can sometimes mimic a nervous system in fight-or-flight state, but more about that later.

Pause to Choose Your Path: Building a Hormone Health Protocol

So far in this book, we've made it clear that you have options when it comes to hormone health. One option that I tossed out, and it's the most commonly utilized, is to go to a conventional doctor's office to be prescribed synthetic hormones. My opinion is that synthetic hormones do a poor job imitating the body's hormones. They're not sourced well; oftentimes, they don't work well; and there are even some scary associations with hormone-sensitive cancers, such as breast cancer or, less commonly, ovarian cancer. The American Cancer Society offers a deep dive into this topic for those who are interested. [9]

Even after tossing out this first option, you still have two clear paths in front of you. Let's first talk about prescribed bioidentical hormone replacement therapy. I want to say this right away: I'm a fan of prescribed BHRT. Typically, the compounding pharmacies that handle these are second to none, when it comes to potency and consistency. If you have a dosage printed on the bottle, that's the dosage you can expect to receive.

I also trust the sourcing of bioidentical hormones, to a much greater extent. They tend to come from high-quality sources. They're in a pure form, and they're highly absorbable, too.

So, what's the catch? Well, you have to go and find a prescribing physician to be your guide. I'm just going to say it—most of these hormone clinics are crazy expensive! I had a patient from Chicago the other day, who told me that just to have one set of lab tests and an annual exam from her doctor, the price tag was $5,000 per year. Yikes.

Here's the thing: In an ideal world, you'd see a prescribing physician for in-depth hormone reviews at least four to six times per year. We have to have respect for the symphony of hormones. Sometimes, they interact in unexpected ways in a very delicate balance, and if you can't adjust on a regular basis, how can you ensure you stay in balance? As lovingly as I can say this, you will be thrown curveballs! What's the plan for when they come?

The other challenging part about finding a physician is locating someone who aligns with your philosophy on hormone therapy. Remember, we've learned why estrogen rarely needs to be prescribed during perimenopause. And yet we see physicians prescribing it all the time.

If you're going to hire a prescribing physician, I recommend referencing WorldLink Medical's list of ABHRT-certified practitioners. This should ensure a number of key principles are understood and embraced.

So, who should go this route? If you have sufficient financial resources and a preference for a managed approach that's reliable but less adaptable, working with a prescribing physician might be the right choice for you.

What's left for everyone else? You have to believe me when I say you're savvy enough to direct the day-to-day of this operation yourself while retaining the regular contact with a primary care physician you already had before beginning. The purpose of this book isn't to trick you into becoming a patient under my care—I really believe you can tackle this yourself, if that is your desire. There may be situations where especially complex needs arise, but most women can take the bull by the horns on their own.

So, that's your third option—taking charge yourself. To state the obvious, it's unlikely that you're a prescribing physician. Your toolkit will not be prescribed BHRT. You will be taking the same principles yet utilizing products that are available over the counter and directly to you. Formulations, delivery methods, potency, and purity have all come so far in the world of dietary supplements. You can get your hands on some really great products that could truly make a splash.

If you choose to go your own way, the name of the game is low and slow. I find that during perimenopause, many women are quite deficient in certain areas, so introducing just a little bit of the key hormones back into the system can go a long way. If you need to fill a massive hole, it might take three months of shoveling to fill it back up. If you filled it back up in three days, that might actually create its own issues.

That's not to say you're bound to taking low dosages. But when you increase them, you do so in a calculated, slow way. Don't make your body process more hormones than it knows what to do with!

Step Four: Begin Introducing Hormone Therapies

We've reached the point in the journey everyone waits for. It's time to begin introducing targeted therapies aimed at bolstering hormone levels. We've learned the complexity involved here. You're likely not just lacking a certain hormone, or having an excess of it, for no reason. There are cofactors, micronutrients, inhibitors, and all kinds of other players in the field to stay mindful of. We have to be wary of how the relevant organs handle the shuttling and clearing of those hormones, as well.

So, it all begs the question: Which hormone do we start with and at what dosage? Before you begin anything, I want to make sure this is well understood: Targeting the hormones with therapy is powerful. You may experience a "bad" symptom right when you begin. Regrettably, many women will throw in the towel immediately when this happens. They will assume that this is actually not for them.

I'm not advocating for continuing if symptoms are dangerous. But if you notice uncomfortable symptoms that aren't inherently dangerous, you should consider it more of a "slow down" signal than a "stop." Respectfully, the hormone pathways we're working with change with age, and introducing hormone therapy can ask a lot of them. It may be that we need to increase or decrease your initial dose until we find a sweet spot.

For some women, a symptom may be an indication of a supportive factor that we need to introduce. For instance, maybe you need to add some magnesium and vitamin B_6 to support your micronutrient levels. I'm not saying to race out and grab a bunch of supplements, but I am saying to stay vigilant. This is where the science and the art of medicine meet. The science says you are this deficient and you need this size of a dosage. The art of medicine may be saying, "Slow down—baby steps. Let's not rush into this."

I can't possibly say it enough—every conversation from here forward makes the assumption that we've completely ditched synthetic hormones. I do not stand behind synthetic hormones for common applications in perimenopause. When we move forward, we do so with the support of biologically identical hormones. I also want to point out that many women would like to think that once the "cellular energy," "drainage," and "nervous system work" boxes have been checked, we can move on to what's more exciting. However, these are boxes that we will always need to work on. Now more than ever, you must continue to support these key areas so that you can get well.

I've spent quite a bit of time trying to introduce the concept that there is no secret sauce or "Easy" button. But let me just say that if there were a secret ingredient, it would be the focus we put on cellular energy, drainage, and the nervous system. My clinic gets better results than many others do in this field because of all the extra attention we give here. Most clinics will jump straight to hormones, but I truly believe that to see optimal results, you have to put in the work on this side of the issue as well.

So, with all those precursors, let's begin the hormone therapy conversation. If you're working with a clinician to prescribe bioidentical hormones, you will ultimately need to find alignment with that individual and follow their protocol. However, the following information provides helpful context so you can bring educated opinions and questions to the table. If you're building your own protocol, I'll help you create an outline.

First things first: Remember that it's worth the wait to introduce one hormone therapy at a time. Doing so allows us to be hyperobservant to how the body responds. We can understand the therapies that make the biggest impact, as well as those that aren't as effective. And so, what we need to do first is to go back to your Ultimate Perimenopause Symptoms Checklist (page 87). Make note of which hormones' checkmarks seem to be stacked in the deficiency column.

Once you've compiled that information, select which hormone you'll begin your journey with. If progesterone is deficient (as is the case for many perimenopausal women), that might be a good place to start. If I could put it in writing right here, I'd give you a recommendation for exactly which product to take. The problem is that science is advancing quickly in this area, and by the time you read this, there might be a new best product to take. However, to compensate for that, use the URL in my Resources section (page 185) to bring you straight to my most up-to-date recommendations. Be sure to check that out periodically after you begin my regimen.

When you begin taking the first hormone, low and slow is the way to go. A little can go a long way. If you know yourself to be someone who reacts strongly to interventions such as this, perhaps start with less of a dosage than is recommended on the side of the bottle. Some people are successful with even a half- or quarter-dosage. Track the exact day you begin—our goal is to complete an entire menstrual cycle of taking just this hormone support before introducing any others.

If your menstrual cycles are long or extremely irregular, aim for a full 30 days before the next product is introduced. Hopefully, things are going well within that first 30 days. Some women will feel great already, whereas others may not see much, if any, result. It can take time to fill those massive potholes, so don't jump to a conclusion that this isn't worthwhile. Remain patient. With most natural therapies and supplements, you'll want to aim for 90 days of consistency before you begin to determine what's working.

And remember, any number of factors may lessen the effectiveness of the hormone therapy you're taking. Before you flat-out stop, you might need to evaluate whether additional support is required to increase the impact. Similarly, it may be that the dosage isn't quite right. You can consider increasing it incrementally.

Another major factor is the product you're taking itself. The nutraceutical (supplement) space has come a long way in just a couple of years. Even 10 years ago, you would be unlikely to see anywhere near the result you could see today by going the nutraceutical route. In this space, the name of the game is absorptivity and delivery method. "Absorptivity" is how well your body can actually absorb the critical components of the product you're taking. "Delivery method," on the other hand, means how those key components are actually delivered into your body.

Take progesterone as an example. Wild yam cream is a popular solution on the market. Remember, wild yams are the original source for many prescribed, compounded bioidentical hormones. If that's the case, the wild yam cream should be a good option, right?

The problem comes down to absorptivity and delivery method. When you put it under a microscope, the progesterone molecules in wild yam cream are so large that it would be difficult for the body to properly absorb them—especially when they're being delivered in the form of a cream applied to the skin. Since much of the product is not immediately absorbed, it ends up rubbing off on your spouse, your pets, your kids, and the rest of your household.

At the time of writing, my favorite progesterone product is also transdermally absorbed by applying it to the skin, similar to the wild yam cream. The important difference? In this product, the size of the progesterone molecule is actually about 100 nanometers—that's smaller than the pores of your skin, allowing for easy absorption. As viewed under a microscope, it's fully absorbed within five minutes. Not bad! See my Resources section (page 185) for the URL that will bring you to this product.

The reason I'm a fan of transdermal application for progesterone is that, once absorbed, it almost immediately enters the lymphatic system and bloodstream. That gives it the opportunity to have a systemic impact very quickly. The company that creates this product I've referenced has also done their own internal research to show that their product is actually 10 times more potent than an oral micronized supplement. That means that, with this product, you can take just a tenth of the dose of the oral product to experience the same results.

Step Five: Layer in Additional Hormone Therapies

I hope you take my advice to layer in hormone therapies one by one. Ideally, some combination of lab results, symptoms, and intuition will have guided you to address your worst deficiency first. If the pothole was large enough, you're very likely still filling it after just 30 days. And yet, this can be a great time to carefully layer in another product. Remember that your end goal is to introduce one new product every 30 days, until you're answering for all of the key deficiencies in your body.

Let's fly through some simple strategies for addressing each of the major hormones at play in perimenopause.

Some hormone replenishment strategies do involve adding dietary supplements to your routine, but I want to make note of this—supplements should not be your only strategy, just as prescribed hormones should not be your only strategy. Success requires the aid of a healthy lifestyle. Take special note of the categories where I have noted lifestyle modifications that trump any supportive product you can take. It may be that you don't need to be taking anything to see improvement, depending on the lifestyle changes you can make.

Progesterone Replenishment

My favorite progesterone product is the transdermal, nano-formulated product we discussed in Step Four. A lot of progesterone products on the market are made from pure sources, but be careful to look beyond that to consider absorptivity and delivery method. If the molecules are too large or the potency is low, even a pure source won't make much impact.

Testosterone & DHEA Replenishment

For testosterone and DHEA, I recommend another nano-formulated product, but this one is taken orally, due to its absorptivity and delivery method—see my Resources section (page 185) for the URL to take you to this product. Note that this formulation also includes a dose of pregnenolone, which, as you may remember from Chapter 2, is the "mother hormone" that plays a vital role—all sex hormones stem from this root.

A good DHEA product should also have ingredients to serve as cofactors for improved absorption.

Thyroid Hormone Replenishment

In the world of thyroid hormones, look for a desiccated beef thyroid product from a reliable source. You want to ensure that this is a grass-fed, pasture-raised product. This may even be worth additional research to understand more about where it's coming from. Ideally, you'll find a brand that runs third-party testing on their lineup, as well.

Melatonin Replenishment

Sex hormones have a monthly cycle, but melatonin has a *daily* cycle. You can supplement melatonin directly, as you probably already know, but I strongly prioritize a bedtime routine and sleep hygiene. Review the tips relating to sleep in Chapter 1, if this is a problem area for you. Don't forget to look to cortisol as well!

Cortisol Balance

Cortisol responds well to adaptogens. Adaptogens are sourced from plants and mushrooms, and they essentially help the body manage stress. You can get adaptogens through your food, in drinks, or as a supplement. Some are more potent than others. Go to the URL in the Resources section (page 185) to learn about optimal products, but I want to state first that nervous system regulation is king in this area.

If you can balance your nervous system, you can spare yourself another item to purchase and keep up with. Work hard on the nervous system regulation tactics we've shared in this book, and you might find that you thrive without cortisol supplementation. Remember, cortisol, like melatonin, has a daily cycle rather than a monthly cycle.

Vitamin D Replenishment

Vitamin D is best replenished by spending more time with the sun on your bare skin . . . for some people. Don't get me wrong, I am a huge fan of getting vitamin D from the sun, first and foremost. Ideally, you should spend at least 20 minutes daily outside in direct sunlight.

But the reality is that many people do not absorb well from the sun alone. Believe it or not, I spent a season of life living in Hawaii, where I had the opportunity to run vitamin D tests with some of the native Hawaiians who'd spent a lifetime outside in the sun. What did I find? Vitamin D deficiency in many cases.

If you are deficient in this vitamin, taking a vitamin D supplement can be beneficial, because supplemental forms contain the necessary cofactors to improve vitamin D absorption. Vitamin D_3 is best absorbed alongside vitamin K_2, so look for the two together. You'll also want to consider how the product is delivered. Many times, it is ideally delivered in a fat state, so you may see such ingredients as olive oil, avocado oil, or similar in your supplement.

Step Six: Evaluate Your Stress

I've said it before, but let me just remind you again—our body can't differentiate between the types of stress it experiences. If you're going through hard things that seem mental, emotional, or spiritual in nature, they can have a greater impact upon your physical health that you might realize. Constantly evaluate your stress and the stressors that surround you. You may be chasing kids, working stressful jobs, in relationships, or otherwise wearing multiple hats.

Do you need support revving up your system? Probably not. What I find is that most women, when asked, would rather have support with settling down and resting. You can take a quality progesterone product, but you should support that choice with the rest of your lifestyle. If you have certain stressors that can be reduced or removed, it might be time to make those moves or cut those ties.

What happens when you can't change the stressors? You can still consider what rest looks like. You can prioritize rest and schedule it into your day. If you catch yourself feeling selfish, ask yourself whether your current state allows you to show up as the best version of yourself *for* yourself, and for others? I challenge you to get to know yourself well enough to understand what it is that settles your system and makes you feel at ease. Everyone understands the concept, but when challenged, many women don't actually know what they would do if they had to take action immediately.

Oftentimes, I observe that my wife struggles to take time for herself because she views attending to our kids and the household as her responsibility and her greatest work. I want to assure you that we don't have a chauvinistic household—everyone else in our home and I are expected to play their role to support the family. And yet many women are inclined to serve others before themselves. That can be beautiful, but you really do need to have the opportunity for rest. You needn't feel apologetic about spending time with your girlfriends or in solitude.

This is a conversation you should feel comfortable having with your partner. If that's not something that comes naturally to you or you have concerns about how your partner would receive it, I have a winning tactic you can use. Say something like this: "I've been reading this book by a guy named Dr. Greg, and he's really emphasizing the importance of having time for rest and solitude. I just want to let you know that this really resonated with me."

Depending on your relationship, there might be some walls coming up as you speak, but here's how you land the plane. "As I was listening to this, I actually realized that neither of us does a good job of finding some time just for ourselves. What I would love to do for us as a couple is to intentionally carve solitude for each of us. So, [dear, babe, bro], what would solitude look like for you?"

Not what they expected to see coming. Be prepared to open yourself up to their answer without getting defensive. There could be any number of things that come to your partner's mind. You might hear about dreams for a weekend away, plans to get back into neglected hobbies, or even just a simple request to have some downtime at home. You might be thinking that they already get a lot more time alone than you've ever experienced, but that's not important right now. Ensure that they feel heard. Help map out what that could look like on your schedule.

Now, hopefully they're mature enough to ask you the same question after you've discussed their answer. If they're not, that's a whole other conversation that's outside the scope of this book. But let's assume they do the decent thing and ask you the same question back. Ensure you've thought through your answer at this point. Maybe you have an eye on abandoned pastimes, unexplored interests, or simply some extra time out with friends. Maybe you want to read a book, take your own weekend away, or who knows what else!

As a husband, I want to honor my bride inside these conversations. Hopefully, your partner wants to do the same.

Step Seven: Incorporate Key Practices into Your Routine

If you are ready to make the most of a healing protocol, there are some little things you can throw on top that will go an incredibly long way. Let's start right at the first thing in the morning. Likely, you roll over and check your phone or scroll social media as soon as you open your eyes. I get that this may help wake you up, but what would the impact be if you took just those first five minutes to practice a breathing exercise? We went over box breathing earlier (see page 28)—try that! Settle your nervous system.

If you're looking for something to dive into right away in the morning, maybe it could be a physical book instead of social media. Maybe you could reach for Scripture or a devotional, a book, or poetry. How different would your day be if you started it off there, instead of falling into the social media pit right away? Just consider those first five minutes as extremely significant for setting the tone for your entire day.

Your morning, in general, shouldn't be crazy sauce. And I get it—you may have kids who need to get to school or you need to leave for work. We can't change some of those realities, but we can plan for them. What are some realistic steps you can take to prevent feeling as if you're going from 0 to 60 in 2.5 seconds? Maybe you need to prep breakfasts for the week ahead or lay out your outfits the night before. Maybe it's time for the kids to make their own breakfasts, if it's age appropriate! Try everything you can to avoid the daily scramble.

Now, here's the part you maybe don't want to hear—try not to drink coffee first thing in the morning. Caffeine will tell your body, "Hey, I've got this!" but it may ultimately cause it to blunt its cortisol response, and that's not a good thing for hormone balance. Holding off for even 30 minutes after waking can make a world of a difference.

Remember, the fundamentals are at play throughout every step. Are you getting nutrients to support your cellular energy? Are you eating enough protein? Are you really trying to slow down to promote nervous system balance? These are the questions you should consistently ask yourself. Just as in any sport, nailing the fundamentals isn't exciting, but it is completely pivotal. By the way, you might be eating "healthy" without eating optimally. Protein is probably the most underrepresented on the average person's plate, so optimize for that, above all else.

What else can you do to support your body? A huge one is helping to promote lymphatic drainage. The lymphatic system is one of the key drainage systems in the body, and it's prone to becoming sluggish. Making routines out of easy two-minute practices goes a long way. Look up some self-massage techniques specifically falling under the banner of "lymphatic massage." You might try tapping, or dry brushing (page 46), too. If you own a rebounding trampoline, hop on there for a few minutes! All of these practices support lymphatic drainage.

The last practices I want you to consider support detoxification. Personal infrared saunas have become more affordable (yet still costly) with the introduction of mobile units. You wouldn't believe the incredible body of research supporting the use of infrared saunas. Consistency could go a long way here. Other options include things like castor oil packs (page 44) or (again) dry brushing.

Remember, you don't need to do every single thing on this list. Maybe you want to try incorporating one practice for detox, one for lymphatic drainage, one for your morning routine, and one for your diet. If it resonates, you might consider adding additional practices or simply staying consistent with what works. If it's not making a huge difference or becomes strenuous, you can switch to something else.

The goal isn't to create an epic wellness routine that has you focused on it day and night. The goal is to get you back to feeling like you again—for you to have to spend less of your mental capacity considering your state of well-being. Hopefully, the symptoms bothering you today fade into distant memory. Hopefully, the routines you do incorporate become almost automatic and a gift to you rather than a burden.

Making Sense of the Seven Steps

With all seven steps in place, work to lay out a sensible protocol that works for you. I'll provide the guardrails, but the exact therapies you use are up to you. Remember to do Step 1 first, evaluating yourself based on your Ultimate Perimenopause Symptoms Checklist (page 87) as well as reviewing your lab test results (if available). You can also use the URL in the Resources section (page 185) to access information about tools, supplements, and more that may be beneficial in your journey.

Evaluate Your Stress (Continually)

Never forget the importance of a nervous system in a state that allows for healing. Nervous system balance was essentially present in Steps Two and Six of our plan for a reason. It's not a quick fix;

it's not "one and done." Purge unnecessary stressors in your life, and for those that are necessary, learn the skill set and the tactics that will help you manage them well.

Energy, Drainage, and Nervous System Balance (Month 1)
This should be your only strategy for at least an entire month. At the end of that month, evaluate the state of your energy and drainage. If you're feeling better faster than you expected, you might be ready to incorporate hormone therapies. If you've noticed you're still bloated, tired, constipated, and frazzled, you might need to go into energy and drainage Month 2.

Incorporate One Hormone Therapy (Month 2)
Without stopping energy, drainage, and nervous system balance work, incorporate your first hormone therapy. If you're going the self-directed route, start low and slow, possibly even at a lower dosage than is recommended on the side of the supplement bottle. If prescribed by a physician, take the dosage they recommend. Continue this one hormone treatment for at least 30 days, or ideally a full menstrual cycle, before introducing additional support.

Incorporate a Second Hormone Therapy (Month 3)
Without stopping what's currently working and necessary, incorporate an additional hormone therapy. Let another month go by as you evaluate how you're feeling. Hopefully, by the end of this month, with two hormone therapies in full swing, you're feeling a lot better. However, remember that deep potholes can take a long time to fill with a shovel. Don't give up!

Add Additional Hormone Therapies & Other Supportive Practices (As Needed)

I never encourage adding more than one hormone therapy at a time. If you find it's necessary to address more hormonal imbalances (for many women, this is common), continue to add them one by one, remembering to go low and slow at first so there's room to ramp up as needed.

The more comfortable you get with the baseline protocol, the more you should look to consider incorporating the key practices addressed in Step Seven that will make massive impacts in small amounts of time. You may be ready to add these right away, or might need time to adjust to all of the changes.

At the end of the day, remember that you're not a supplement or a prescription away from optimal wellness. These can be invaluable components, but a true health routine is comprehensive. If you consider your lifestyle, would it now appear healthy if you took away the supplement or the prescribed product?

I don't like throwing people under the bus for diet. You may actually eat well and work out regularly! And yet things like stress, underlying chronic infection, and yes, even perimenopause can reveal some of the ways in which our lifestyle is not conducive to our overall health and well-being. Keep up with the State of the Union exercise as you go, so you can have a pulse on this. It's time to start thriving again!

5.
ONE SIZE DOESN'T FIT ALL: MAKING MICRO-ADJUSTMENTS

You probably jumped into the previous chapter with excitement. Finally, time to take the bull by the horns! But as a protocol comes together and the first month or two on it goes by, different questions arise: How am I supposed to feel now? Is this not working? Am I impatient? Am I doing something wrong? This seems to be working, but how long do I keep doing this?

We'll tackle questions like these in the current chapter. A perimenopause protocol is fluid, just like perimenopause itself. As you move forward, I'll introduce you to a toolkit for making the necessary adaptions that keep you moving in the right direction for the long term. Most women start noticing positive changes fairly quickly after they've introduced a comprehensive protocol. I hope you're one of them. If you're not, just know that you aren't broken or beyond repair. There are other women in your shoes—they finally start the protocol that *should* work, but they don't see that quick result they'd expected. We'll help you respond appropriately!

What to Do When Nothing's Changing

You started up a perimenopause protocol. Nothing's changed . . . at all. Nothing seems particularly worse, but nothing seems to be improving, either. You're probably wrestling with how long you should continue on before making what could be necessary changes to your protocol. Most people are concerned about being impatient (which is very possible, too).

Here's my first question: Did you skip chapters in this book? If you made straight for the hormone chapter or the protocol-building chapter, then you might be guilty of being impatient and reaping the rewards of it. And, hey, we've all done that at times. Grace to you. But I'd encourage you to go back and understand the method to this madness. The foundational work isn't here to fill pages; it's actually essential to making the rest of this work.

I understand a lot of hormone clinics will tell you this can all be solved by just taking a few hormones. It's really not that simple for most women. You cannot skip the energy, drainage, and nervous system work that prepares your body to take hormone therapies in stride.

On the other hand, if you've stuck with me this far, having honored drainage and cellular energy, and done the necessary nervous system work, you've supplied the necessary support to your body and tracked your progress in these areas. All of that is good. But now you've started taking something that's supposed to support your hormones and you're wondering when you'll see results.

Every woman is different. My earnest hope for you is that you'll quickly see the results you're looking for. But I want to prepare you to stick with your initial protocol for at least three to four months before you can properly determine whether it isn't working (if that becomes the case, we have tools for that, too). Continue to put in the foundational work, take the first hormone therapy product for at least a month, add the next when you've mapped that out, and pay close attention to how you feel along the way. We're looking for 90 to 120 days of consistency before we can determine that, yes, tweaks need to be made.

Why so long? The worse your foundations were when you started (not draining well, being completely fatigued or totally frazzled), the longer it will take just to reach baseline in those areas. And as we've discussed, if you're less than optimal in these areas, it will slow the rest of the work. In case you were wondering, foundational work is never done. As nervous system regulation, cellular energy, and drainage improve, you may be able to move certain supplementary supports to an as-needed basis. You might even begin to rotate products in and out in a cycle so you can continue experiencing the benefits of each. But you're never done—you have to stay vigilant because once the foundation cracks, everything is at risk of tumbling down.

Foundational work aside, the time it takes to see success depends on how large your hormone deficiency was. The bigger the pothole, the more shoveling we need to do to backfill all of the dirt. And that's okay! Have some grace for yourself in the journey.

One final thing to consider: If you did lab testing, how did the rest of your markers look? I had a woman come into my clinic the other day with hormones that were nowhere near optimal. She also had a liver enzyme panel done and discovered that her liver enzymes were five times higher than where we wanted them to be. Think about that—five times higher. In cases like these, is it really as simple as blaming the hormones?

By the way, your body isn't Amazon Prime®. You didn't get to where you are overnight, and you can't get out of it overnight! So, use that three- to four-month time period to make an evaluation of whether any progress is being made. If not, the rest of this chapter can help you troubleshoot.

A Note about Personal Care

This book wasn't written to fill up my own clinic, or clinics belonging to friends of mine. My hope and prayer for anyone reading this book is that you can use the tools we've outlined to be successful with managing your own ongoing care or being a more knowledgeable collaborator with the practitioner of your choice.

But I'd be remiss if I didn't mention the possibility of an extremely complex case. Just because things haven't "clicked" in your journey yet doesn't mean you're a complex case. However, I have seen a handful of cases that just did better under managed care. Severe mold toxicity, underlying non-alcoholic fatty liver disease, Lyme disease, and the most stubborn cases of insulin resistance have come into my clinic, and I think that having a knowledgeable advocate is beneficial and worthwhile for people in these situations.

So, take your time to troubleshoot. Try to be patient with yourself and the journey—go through the rest of this chapter, to start! But if no amount of troubleshooting brings any success, there's no shame in contacting a trusted practitioner to get hands-on support. Nothing you did was wasted; it only made you more knowledgeable about being your own best advocate.

Be Responsive to Your Cycle

If you're just not seeing the improvements you were looking for, one thing you can experiment with is altering your dosage of progesterone in accordance with your menstrual cycle. All women inherently understand that the cycle shifts massively throughout the course of a month, but not all women honor that reality. As you go along, you may want to consider utilizing the Ultimate Perimenopause Symptoms Checklist (page 87) multiple times throughout the month. You might be able to pinpoint whether your symptoms surge during particular parts of your cycle.

During the luteal phase (just after ovulation), many women can benefit from an increased intake of progesterone that's greater than the baseline dosage they take throughout the rest of the month. It may be well worth considering.

Be Honest About Your Stress

If you find yourself caught in an extremely stressful job, relationship, or other life circumstance, that constant state of stress is going to trump everything else you're trying to do. If that's you, have some grace for yourself. But at this point, it might be time to sit with yourself and ask this question: "If I were my own clinician and I had to determine what it is that could be preventing these hormones from doing what they're designed to do, what would I determine that could be?"

Sit with that question for a bit. If financial stress, marital stress, or specific scenarios come to mind, you may have your answer. I spoke to a woman once who had to go through the pain and emotion of kicking a problematic adult child out of her house. She probably hadn't considered the impact that strained relationship and that decision were having on her physical health. But when I spoke to her six weeks later, she and her family were thriving. She felt that she had the bandwidth to take this on. She was sleeping better and at ease.

What is that for you? Is there something that needs to be addressed in your life that could greatly impact your mental and physical health? Not every problem has an obvious solution, but if there's something that needs to come to the forefront, let it take precedence! Work with a professional, if needed. Don't ignore the sources of stress that hold you back.

What to Do if You Feel Worse than Ever

If you started this protocol and found in some amount of time that you actually feel worse than ever, you might be thinking that this just isn't for you. If you had a severe reaction to something, I do encourage you to reach out to your regular doctor or contact emergency services. For the vast majority who had the general feeling of being "off," I need you to know something: Sometimes, the body reacts before it responds. Oof. Not what most of us want to hear.

Maybe you suddenly have hot flashes or your cycles seem to have gotten worse. I'll be honest—just like you, I don't love that. I'm not trying to pretend that symptoms are fun, because they're not. But what I am telling you is that it doesn't mean your body is wrong. Your first step is to pinpoint why you feel worse. What exactly feels wrong? What are the new symptoms you're experiencing?

Is there new fatigue? Mood swings? Skin reactions? All of these symptoms could be caused by the hormone therapy interacting with your drainage pathways. If this is you, you might want to consider doing some deeper detox work.

Remember that, earlier, we discussed the key organs that take a part in this process. Certain symptoms may indicate that your liver and gut are straining to keep up with the work you're trying to do. In these cases, a deeper look at how your gut and liver are functioning in general might be warranted. You might need to consider additional support for these organs after looking at symptoms, lab test results, or both. Previously, these hormones were profoundly depleted; now, you're introducing more and the organs are being asked to step up their game! That's not trivial—they need to get back to work and they might protest because of it!

Even nutrient depletion is a factor. Your body could be crying out for essential micronutrients that you're lacking. Perhaps you need to add magnesium or other quality minerals to your regimen to start feeling improvement.

Whew. This might be hard to hear, because suddenly things sound more complicated. I know you desperately want to feel well, and that's what I want for you as well. But in that pursuit, I need you to know that you could be making progress even if you're feeling worse. When you're feeling worse, you're at least getting valuable feedback from your body that suggests you're tapping into something. If you feel nothing is different at all, it's harder to determine your next steps. Obviously, though, this isn't where we want to stay. You need to get curious. You may need to make adjustments, but you do not need to panic. Try not to just use the word "worse." To be actionable: You have to be able to define what's worse and when it's worse, if you want to move forward.

Oh, and in case you're that person who went ahead and jumped on multiple hormone therapies all at once, you may have your answer there. Start with one! This is an ultramarathon, not a 100-yard dash. Slow down, track your treatment, and tweak it along the way. Be invested enough to do the microtuning that will have the major impact.

Forming Your Plan B

We've discussed how hormone deficiencies are like potholes in the road—some are deeper than others. If you've been patient but still ultimately determine that your plan A isn't working, you might be that person who needs to take the next step. My hope for you is that you've done due diligence, that you've stayed consistent, you've made the microadjustments, you've even incorporated some of the additional support that you felt your body may need.

But at the end of the day, if the needle still isn't moving, it's unavoidable that certain people—maybe 10 percent or less—will need to strongly consider the route of managed care. This book wasn't written to trick you into getting a little bit of the secret sauce and saving the rest for the moment you decide to come work with a professional. My philosophy is to "sell the farm." Without knowing you and your exact circumstances, I'm providing as much information as possible here in this book, to support you in your journey.

And yet, sometimes when we manage our own care, there's a risk of being so far inside the jar that we can't read the label. In times like these, a new perspective may be beneficial. That someone could guide you and ask good questions that you may not have even considered. If you've held out, maybe that first step is running comprehensive lab tests so you can have a better sense of what you're up against. Or it may just be that you should consider aligning with a health coach and practitioner who can provide you with support for the long run.

Just so you know, you're not alone. Reach out—my team and I would be happy to offer you support in any way we can. It may just be that there are factors at play that complicate your case, and that's okay.

"Nothing Works for Me"

If you've uttered this statement and if it's rung true, you need to know you haven't gotten to the bottom yet. I hold the firm belief that our body was designed to heal. Our body is always seeking a state of homeostasis. Are there complex cases? Oh, yes. There can be genetic roadblocks, such as the MTHFR mutation, toxic loads, chronic infection, trauma . . . Do those have an impact on this healing process? One hundred percent.

Recently, a patient who entered my practice had been chronically ill for probably decades. Once she started working with me and my team, she actually started to feel better quite quickly. It looked like a huge win for everyone. But then, she began to drink. It was as if the brakes were squealing as her healing journey rushed to a halt.

At this point, she came to me and said, "I don't think this is working for me." I had the opportunity at this point to slow down, back up, and make some observations. I said, "What I observed is that you said you were feeling better." She adamantly agreed, so I continued. "What it sounded like is that you started to drink for whatever reason, and then things shifted." She agreed again.

There's a part of you that gets used to being unhealthy. Whether you know it or not, you may have conditioned the people around you to respond to your current state of health. Maybe you get special treatment, maybe you miss invitations because they assume you are unable to participate... There are endless possibilities, depending on how it is that you've presented yourself.

So, even though in your head you want to be well, you don't even know what "well" is like. Maybe a part of you is saying that you're used to chaos and being unhealthy, so perhaps it's safest to stick with what you know.

In the case of this patient, we had a heavy conversation about this. We both cried a little bit. What I ultimately said to her was that this felt like sabotage. I told her that maybe she was subconsciously afraid that, once she got healthy, she'd face uncertainty: What would be expected of her? Would people still love her well? It was the unknown.

Let's set this in a more familiar context. Take a marriage where one spouse was raised in a stable, loving home; the other was raised in chaos—fighting, bickering, stress... Both of these partners have a learned idea of what a normal household looks like. There's clearly a "right" and "wrong," but that doesn't matter. Your experience unconsciously teaches you which is "normal."

So, what happens? Even though the partner raised in stress and dysfunction has something deep inside them that craves stability and peace, it's uncomfortable to experience it! In many cases, we see this partner reintroduce what's familiar and comfortable—fighting and chaos. It doesn't feel right, but it feels normal.

If you're this person, my heart goes out to you. I love you, and I want to see you get well. You're worthy of feeling well. Have you sat down to have a hard conversation with yourself yet? Yes, you want to get well, but do you feel that you truly deserve it? Do you worry about how others will respond? Will they still love you if you become well and don't require extra attention?

You're not broken. Your body is waving caution flags, not surrender flags. Get curious—listen deeper, not louder. A lot of people just want to throw up their hands and say nothing works for them, or that they're always the exception. Let's not live in the mindset that this brings. Sometimes, what's not working tells us exactly where to look next.

I have five kids. When I hear such words as *nothing, always,* and *never*, I'm going to challenge it every time. "*Nothing* works for you?" Usually, the challenge brings in an answer like, "Well... not *nothing.*"

Beware the self-talk and the impact it can have. When a woman came into my clinic once, together we unveiled an absolutely wild ride that no doctor or clinician had ever gone through with her. We talked about the time her house flooded and it led to mold exposure. We talked about likely Lyme disease exposure, a 15-year run on birth control, and more. She had some of the craziest stomach issues, she couldn't gain weight . . . it was eye-opening for both of us!

But when I asked her how she felt, at the end of the conversation, she said, "Skeptical." My response to her was this: "I hear you. That has to be a tough place to be." She felt that she was just being a realist. There's something to that. She, like others, has probably tried things. She probably had optimism in each of them until, one by one, nothing ended up being the solution she hoped for.

And yet, imagine the damage this mindset can do when you set out on a journey. If you don't have any faith that you'll reach your destination, you probably won't. Again, you're worthy of getting better. Work on truly believing that! If you have someone who cares for you deeply, train them to support you so you don't have to shoulder this alone.

By the way, if that person is a man, you might be worried that bringing him in means getting his unsolicited advice and attempts to fix things. Here's how to avoid that. Simply ask him whether he can ask you these two questions every single day:

1. What's better?

2. How can I help?

The first question is not "How are you?" If your spouse asks that question, you might feel that you have to ask them to sit down and buckle up for a marathon of "this hurts, this sucks, this isn't right." And, by the way, we don't need to pretend that the symptoms aren't there! But when we direct ourselves to look for the one thing that's better, we train ourselves to notice it more. When we focus on noticing it, we benefit immensely.

As for the second question, I always tell my female patients this: Men are like dogs (sorry, guys). When you need help with something, it's completely okay and beneficial to be abundantly clear. Make sure you give an objective definition of what "done" looks like and describe what completing it successfully looks like. Once it's accomplished, a proverbial pat on the head will send him back for more. Men are fixers! Feeling that we have some ability to help in the midst of everything you're going through will, hopefully, go a long way for both you and your spouse.

By the way, you might have a spouse who's such a fixer that it actually turns to frustration. I'm not justifying it, but perhaps it helps bring context to the situation: He wants to help solve your problem and has no idea how to do so. So, what happens next? Frustration builds. It's not directed at you, but it can feel like it at times. If there are ways that he can genuinely support you in any meaningful way, let him know!

By the way, ladies: If there's a part of you that, when asked these questions, says, "Nothing's better, and I don't want your help," I'd ask you to check with yourself on that. Check your heart! Where is that coming from? Do you feel unworthy of being served? Do you feel that there will be an obligatory response, or that this will turn into a favor for a favor? Try to disregard those feelings.

Allow yourself to be served. Many people struggle with this. It could be a whole weekend seminar, but I'll leave you with the simple challenge—allow yourself to be served!

When to Overhaul

If it's time to completely overhaul your wellness protocol, you won't wonder whether it is. The only time to overhaul is when something is fundamentally wrong. If you were building a house and the foundation itself was crooked, you'd be forced to overhaul. In all other scenarios, you can rebuild individual sections.

Build Your Toolbox

When things just don't go as planned, where do you turn? Hopefully this book has introduced you to the concept of really listening to your body. Maybe you're even able to pick up on signs that your liver is performing suboptimally, or that you're frazzled and running on high cortisol throughout your day. I would love for you to be able to process the signals your body is sending you and then take action.

But when you're driving and see a warning light come onto your car's dashboard, interpreting the meaning is only half the battle. What do you actually do about it? The reality is that *this for that* medicine won't get you where you want to go. Seeking out the next silver bullet for every new symptom is something I strongly urge you to avoid doing. Instead, commit to building a toolbox.

In that toolbox, you might have certain tactics, supplements, or ideas, but your goal is to stick to them, rather than falling for the latest TikTok video with new and novel information. Trust me when I say there has yet to be an example where the result lives up to the claim made in the video you watch. It's not that these tools don't work at times, but nothing in and of itself is your silver bullet. You're looking for those 100 golden BB pellets.

So, let's build the toolkit that you can stick with and turn to when things just aren't going well. Remember that the State of the Union exercise (page 24) and the Ultimate Perimenopause Symptoms Checklist (page 87) are your friends—use them to help determine what it is that might be off and prohibiting further progress.

Nervous System Tools

You're a veteran now, and you probably knew we would be starting here. Your nervous system toolkit allows you to prep your figurative job site. You can't use a power drill effectively without inserting a bit, and you can't heal without priming your nervous system. There are tools that can help. I want to suggest this one first: Maybe you need to talk to a professional. If you've already been dutifully employing some of the tactics introduced in this book but just aren't seeing your stress levels decrease, you may need to honor your nervous system by getting more help.

Mental health therapists are equipped with de-escalation capabilities, and can help you learn to process stress when it can't be avoided. I can't emphasize enough the impact that this can have on your mental and physical health. By the way, you might have the opportunity to unpack things that you've left completely unprocessed. In many cases, that alone may help settle your system.

What are the other tools to come back to? Breathwork is one. Box breathing (page 28) is a simple version that can be used on a routine basis, but others, such as breath holding and forced exhalation, can be extremely helpful as well.

Cellular Energy Tools

Cellular energy is like the batteries that put the "power" in "power tools." Go back to your nutrition. Ask yourself honestly whether you're still getting enough water, protein, and fatty acids. If you haven't, consider jumping onto a mitochondrial support supplement (for my suggestions, go to the URL in the Resources section (page 185). Your cells do actually respond very well to high-quality nutritional support, so a supplement can be key.

For more information on supporting cellular energy, jump all the way back to Chapter 1 in this book.

Gut-Support Tools

In our drainage funnel, our gut sits at the bottom. As we get older, the parietal cells in our stomach, designed to produce acid, become less efficient. Put simply, that means you might need a little extra support for your digestive process. If your digestion is off, it can be very uncomfortable. Plus, it could clog the entire drainage funnel. And as we've already discussed, that can put cracks in the foundation of your entire healing protocol.

Some people have success with gentle products, such as digestive enzymes or bitters. Depending on how significant your digestive issues are, you might even want to supplement something as strong as hydrochloric acid (checking with your health-care provider first about a suitable product, and the form to purchase it in), if the bitters or enzymes fail to help you. The goal is to take some of the burden off of the gut.

Liver-Support Tools

I'm a big fan of providing extra support to the liver—so much so that we already provided a number of tools for that (see page 45). At that time, we very briefly made mention of glutathione. Glutathione is one of the most potent antioxidants available in supplemental form. Regrettably, it can be poorly absorbed in an average dietary supplement product. An IV is probably the most absorbable way to get glutathione into your system, but it's also outrageously expensive.

These days, there are some over-the-counter supplements that have formulated glutathione capsules to be optimal for delivery. Be mindful of this when selecting a product. A liposomal glutathione might go a lot farther than others.

Other Tools

One very helpful and simple tool is a tracking journal. Write down all of your symptoms (and everything else) that you're experiencing, and continue to note any updates. When people tell us a few months down the road that they're not feeling better, my first response is to send them to their tracking journal or the State of the Union exercise (page 24) that they completed—9.5 times out of 10, this person will discover they've come a lot farther than they realized. You forget, faster than you might think, how rock bottom felt! It can be frustrating to feel that you didn't even notice the changes as they happened, but it's a good encouragement to stay aware.

Beyond your symptoms, consider tracking your menstrual cycles, your poop (yes, really), your food, and your mood. Start to pull in other data points that could make sense with the symptoms you're having.

Have a bodily movement toolkit as well! What makes sense for you? For me, walking is the tool I've found, to go outside, get moving, and keep my joints healthy.

By the way, as you look through all of these potential tools that are available to you, I continue to encourage you not to try six of them all at one time. Incorporate them one at a time. Stick with what works and don't stress about what doesn't.

Maybe you need to add simple things to your toolkit: Do you need to have date nights with your spouse or spend some time with your girlfriends? Do you need to go get your nails done or sit down with a coffee somewhere? Many times, when we consider wellness protocols, we jump to cold plunges, biohacking, and infrared therapy. We look for advanced methodologies and crazy protocols. But how are you supporting your basic needs? How are you doing mentally, emotionally, and even socially?

Other lifestyle tools you might want to look for are:
- Castor oil packs (page 44)
- Vibration plate
- Dry brushing (page 46)
- Rebounding
- Infrared sauna (page 134)
- Red light therapy

Many of these tools support drainage in different ways. Some offer an extra oomph to the liver, and some are versatile in terms of the support they offer. Find which ones resonate best with you and your needs! The idea is to support your system, not simply suppress symptoms.

The toolbox exists for cases where things feel as if they're heading in the wrong direction. Instead of spiraling, you go to your toolbox and deduce which drawer you need to pull out and grab something from. It's not about always sustaining every single one of these practices; it's about intelligently determining which one you can benefit from most when things hit the fan.

Chasing the Wrong Cause

If you're one of those people who has hyperanalyzed your Ultimate Perimenopause Symptoms Checklist (page 87) to no end, you're well aware of how much overlap exists among some of the key symptoms. For instance, it can be hard to determine the source of fatigue when there are so many potential causes. At some point, you might have to ask yourself if you've fallen for an imitator.

I've had countless firsthand experiences with this. Women come to our clinic after washing out on a hormone clinic's protocol that just didn't work. The hormone clinic told them they just needed large doses of these three hormones and they'd do great! When they didn't, they sought out further support.

Let's go through some of the key issues behind this.

Misdiagnoses & Common Imitators

There are red herrings that often end up chased down within a health protocol. Unfortunately, that often means the real cause is left unnoticed and unaddressed. Let's look at a few.

Fatigue

Common Misdiagnosis: Low estrogen and low testosterone

Potential Missed Causes: Underlying low-level anemia, vitamin B_{12} deficiency, stress hormones off

Is it possible that low estrogen and low testosterone are causing symptoms of fatigue? Yes. However, sometimes a deeper cause can be missed, and one I see often is underlying low-level anemia. This is where we have to go back to the conversation of lab tests' reference ranges versus optimal health ranges. I like to see the lab test result's value for hemoglobin, found on a complete blood count (CBC) between 13.5 and 14.5. If you were to look at a lab's reference range, it will allow for a much wider range of numbers before they'd ever call someone anemic. That's why I specifically use the term *low-level* anemia. It might not be diagnosable, but that doesn't mean it's optimal. And if it's not optimal, it's likely contributing to fatigue.

Vitamin B_{12} deficiency is another possibility. This is fairly straightforward, but again we have to consider a functional perspective on lab tests. We're looking for optimal B_{12}, not just B_{12} that's "in range."

The final possibility is that we need to look at the hypothalamic-pituitary-adrenal axis. That's a lot of long words to describe the primary system that controls your body's response to stress. Think of your stress hormones, such as cortisol, DHEA, and cortisone. These are most accurately measured in a diurnal (daytime) pattern. If you haven't tested them, it might be worth considering whether fatigue is among your biggest concerns.

Weight Gain & Weight-Loss Resistance

Common Misdiagnosis: Hypothyroidism

Potential Missed Causes: Insulin resistance or cortisol dysregulation

This is an interesting symptom, because three of the key hormones discussed in this book could be at the source. In my experience, most women experiencing weight-loss resistance have it in their head that a sluggish thyroid is to blame. That can be true in some cases, but what I've found is that two other extremely likely culprits are insulin resistance (cells have become resistant to insulin) or cortisol dysregulation.

If you've been going to war with hypothyroidism but haven't addressed insulin or cortisol, that could be something to consider if your protocol is stalling out!

Anxiety or Irritability

Common Misdiagnosis: Low progesterone

Potential Missed Causes: Gut inflammation or histamine intolerance

This is not to discount anxiety or irritability caused by the state of your mental health. However, if a woman intuitively identifies that these symptoms appear to be tied to hormones, low progesterone tends to be the first place she or her practitioner should look at. Low progesterone can absolutely be a source of anxiety or irritability, but if you're not seeing the needle move when addressing it, it could be possible that you're up against gut inflammation or histamine intolerance. We find that women who experience histamine intolerance especially find their bodies to be in a highly reactive state or even a state of alert.

Hot Flashes & Night Sweats

Common Misdiagnosis: Low estrogen

Potential Missed Causes: Blood sugar instability

Hot flashes and night sweats are among the most famous menopause or perimenopause symptoms. Because of this, most will jump to assume that low estrogen is at the source. That can be true, especially in menopause. If it occurs during perimenopause, on the other hand, I've made other interesting observations. A number of the women who see me at my clinic have utilized continuous glucose monitors. What we've found is that many of them make their most impactful nutrition choices in the evening, right before bed.

The result? Blood sugar crashes going into bedtime, causing a hot flash.

Breast Tenderness & Breast Fullness

Common Misdiagnosis: Estrogen dominance

Potential Missed Causes: Poor liver detox or exposure to endocrine-disrupting chemicals

Although estrogen dominance can be a cause for the feeling of breast tenderness or fullness, poor liver detox can actually be a common issue as well. If the liver's work is sluggish, there are major implications for estrogen, too, so it can be a chicken-and-the-egg scenario.

I've also found that endocrine-disrupting chemicals, which are often present in personal or household products, can be at the source of this. By mimicking real estrogens, these xenoestrogens (fake estrogens) can have systemic impact.

Keep it Simple

It's true, there's no recipe card. You can't grab the "hot flash" card and find the one thing you should take that will make the problem go away. But what you do have is a toolbox. Consider this akin to building a birdhouse in a woodshop. If you've never done it before, you might have a sense for which tool to use at which point in the process, but there could very well be times when it's unclear which tool to use. You might even find that everyone tells you to do one thing, only to discover it works better to go another way.

As much as I'd love for you to have a recipe box, the toolbox is the best offer. The human body is extremely complex, but that shouldn't be discouraging. Would you rather hit a dead end and feel that you have no additional options, or know that you can simply turn back and take another route?

If your initial protocol doesn't go as swimmingly as you'd hoped, that's when you can consider individual areas that could benefit from a modified approach. Maybe you've been targeting low estrogen when you need to focus a little more on your liver. Maybe you've neglected the role of your gut or blamed the thyroid for cortisol's problem.

I need you to know that my clinic's success rate is very high, because we've spent over 20 years refining these protocols. Before you get overwhelmed, bring yourself back to the fundamentals: energy, drainage, and nervous system regulation, which lead you to hormone therapy, stress management, and the other lifestyle recommendations introduced in Chapter 4.

Even with curveballs, the game hasn't changed and these fundamentals are still your fallback. Almost all of the "imitators" or "missed causes" we just went through relate directly back to energy, drainage, stress, and hormones. The tricky part is identifying which is the culprit for which symptom.

And yes, in some cases other nutritional support is beneficial (as in the case of B_{12}). Thankfully, these are simple additions to a protocol, and we connect you with recommendations in the Resources section (page 185).

6.
KEYS FOR LONG-TERM SUCCESS

Wow, we've almost made it to the end of this book. My hope for you is that you have a protocol in place. If you're a quick reader, maybe the jury's still out and you're waiting to see what works. If you're more methodical, maybe you're here and you already know some of what's working and what isn't. In any case, I hope you stay committed to finding your groove. This is not one-size-fits-all, but between all of the tools, tactics, and tricks shared in this book, my hope and prayer is that every reader will benefit.

So, the question on your mind might be something like this: What now? What's the endgame? As much as you can find your rhythm and gain power over perimenopause, what about menopause itself, which is looming up ahead? We're going to do a deep dive in this chapter. The goal here will be to tie up loose ends and help you to set up a successful, gentle transition into menopause when the time comes.

The End Goal

Let me state something we (hopefully) all know: Perimenopause can be a lengthy period in a woman's life. It can last for years—sometimes, even a decade! That probably brings up a question: If a protocol works, do we ride with it until the end of perimenopause? Here's the good news and bad news: There are evolutions to this. The protocol you create is not static and should be viewed as completely adaptable to suit your needs.

The reality is that the endgame is metabolic and hormonal resilience. Put simply, I want you to feel that you're in control! One patient once came to me and said, "Dr. Greg, I used to follow this diet and do these exercises and have a predictable result, but now I feel like I'm out of control." I want you to gain that control back by understanding the tools you have in front of you.

If I were to break it down, metabolic resilience consists of control of your metabolic hormones, including insulin, vitamin D, and the thyroid hormones. I would define "hormonal resilience," on the other hand, by how you feel: Do you feel resilient, settled, and driven? Are you motivated? Is your libido back? Do you feel like every bit of the woman you want to be?

In time, I hope the foundational work becomes less like work and more like an automation. In time, such things as sleep hygiene, promoting drainage, nervous system regulation, gut health, and blood sugar control should come more naturally . . . so long as you've made some of the necessary lifestyle changes.

Your hormones are supported with precision, but I also want to be transparent with you: This is living, breathing, and ultimately, a moving target. Your body is designed to make a slow and gentle transition into menopause at some point, and that forward march means your hormones will be impacted in different ways along the way. Finally, as you enter menopause, your ovaries will come to the point where they essentially cease production of estradiol.

If we plan for it, you won't be caught off guard and floundering when it happens. I recently had a conversation with a woman who went into menopause without a baseline or an understanding of what she was moving into. She just told me that the wheels fell off. She didn't feel prepared, and her life was full of stress. I won't get into the details, but suffice to say that she was dealing with more extreme stress, condensed into a short period of time, than many of us will encounter in a lifetime.

Even though the stress felt sudden, we looked back: We reviewed everything she had gone through even before this time, to determine how her "rain bucket" had filled up to the brim over time. You might or might not know this, but as perimenopause advances toward menopause, your adrenal glands are actually designed to accelerate. The body essentially says, "Chop, chop. Time to pick up the pace."

The problem and risk for women, such as this client of mine, is that everything that's happened up until this point in their life can mean that there's risk the adrenal glands have already tapped out by the time they get to menopause. A lot of contributors can be at play, chiefly stress. To continue using the example of the woman I worked with: On top of all that she went through later in life, she had had an extremely challenging childhood. If you haven't looked into adverse childhood experiences (ACEs) and can relate, some research is well worth your time.

No wonder why a belly flop into the deep end of menopause pushed this poor woman into losing all control. My hope for you, the reader, is that we're doing the necessary work to set the stage and prevent this kind of experience. When you go into menopause, metabolic and hormonal resilience will be the reins on the horse, and will give you some control.

What to Do When Your Protocol "Kind of" Works

In Chapter 5, we did a deep dive into troubleshooting your protocol. But I want to come back to this topic one last time. Picture yourself sitting at a control board full of knobs and levers. Each and every one of us sit in this figurative chair when overseeing our health.

The problem is that most of the devices turn things up and down without our understanding much about the impact we experience.

More than anything, I hope that this book served as an owner's manual for that control board. I hope you learned a bit about the key controls and what happens when you dial one up or down. Maybe you haven't committed everything to memory, and that's okay. You can always come back to this book as your reference.

If the key hormones, drainage, cellular energy, and nervous system regulation are some of the key dials that get moved up and down frequently, what are some of the dusty knobs way off in the corner that could be tweaked just a bit to provide some extra benefit?

Micronutrients

Could there be fine-toothed micronutrient deficiencies inside your body? Each is of the utmost importance to our bodily functions. I just read one piece of research doubling down on the profound impact of a vitamin A deficiency on our health and well-being. That's just one of the numerous micronutrients needed by our body. Remember that the micronutrients are essentially the letter vitamins, plus the key minerals.

Sometimes, micronutrient deficiencies mean you need to make a dietary tweak. Other times, a supplement will give an extra oomph.

Blaming Success

This is more of a mindset element. We had a woman at our practice who was taking a DHEA product to increase her testosterone. It worked! But in the process of that, she experienced a sudden bout of cystic acne. What would your response be? If you're like most, you'd probably say, "Abandon ship!" That's how she felt. She told me there's no way she should be going through this again at her age.

And I agree! But we have to ask this: Why would experiencing an optimal level of testosterone cause cystic acne? When we dug deeper, we found that her basophils (a white blood cell differential found in a CBC lab test) were elevated. One potential cause for elevated basophils is having a high number of parasites in the body.

Guess what one of the symptoms can be? We backed up together and went back through this work so that her body could support the optimal level of testosterone.

By the way, this woman had actually done work to address parasites years earlier. Remember that very few things are" one and done" with our body. Sometimes, you have to go back for round two! Be careful of considering yourself to be "already past that." Especially when you deal with pathogens and toxins, you have to remember you're not hermetically sealed in a sterile environment. We live in a stressful society filled with toxins and chemicals—sometimes, new exposures reverse some of our progress!

Circadian Rhythm

Circadian rhythm brings us back to the sleep hygiene conversation. Most of us know circadian rhythm as the course of a day. We intuitively get that there are waking hours and sleeping hours. What we don't often acknowledge is that we can play tricks on our body by screwing with it. Blue light exposure is a sort of epidemic these days. If you find yourself staring at phones and computer screens all day, especially late into the night, you're confusing your body!

Is your morning routine out of control and crazy? Is it at all possible to make some changes, to have some time to ease into the day? An incredible body of research has been done to show just how much impact improper circadian rhythm can have on our health. We're talking about literally shortening your life span! Don't make this simple mistake.

Filtering Health Trends

Wow, are there some fancy, crazy health trends out there. If you know your TikTok eras, this will date the book, but at the time I write this, it seems that everyone's talking about peptide therapy, saunas, PEMF mats, and vibration plates, among other things. You can fill in the trend with whatever you see going around you right now.

Here's the thing—I'm a fan of advanced therapies! There are times that it makes sense to have at them! But this comes with a caveat: So many people coming into my practice are virtually tackling all of the trends—yet, they still feel like garbage. Don't fall for the hype that would have you believe in an instant cure or an "Easy" button. If an advanced therapy really resonates with you, maybe incorporate it while keeping your perspective.

Also, know that the right thing at the wrong time is still the wrong thing. Think about detox, for example. I see people all the time who do long-term detox. Your body cannot handle doing detox for weeks at a time! Think of yourself as an underwater diver without external oxygen. Eventually, that diver needs to come up for air, and so does your body. It's okay to take breaks!

Self-Talk During Breaks

My last point drives me right into this one. You may urgently need to slow down and take a break. But when you do, what happens to your self-talk? Some women feel that they've screwed up everything and they need to start over. Others feel like a failure and simply give up. By the way, some people even unknowingly sabotage themselves! We talked about that more in the previous chapter.

As you start to feel better, keep your head on a swivel. If you can't take a simple break to recharge and come back to your health protocol with a new invigoration, check your heart. What kind of thoughts are running through your brain? Do you have the ability to look back and admire your progress, or do you get caught up worrying about the progress you haven't made and the pauses you take?

If you're in that second category, you need to reevaluate. It's really tough to feel that you should keep going if you doubt the benefit. Don't let yourself get there.

Set It and Forget It

Let's use the example of a control board one more time. You might have experienced running something resembling one, for work or as a volunteer. If not, you can probably still picture the scene. In many cases, these giant boards contain literally a hundred or more dials, levers, gauges, and buttons. And yet, many look more intimidating than they really are.

Let's use an audio board as an example. During a live music production, a giant audio board is the master control for the way a crowd will experience a show. Some of these dials require constant adjustment to ensure the sound is right. That's why an entire sound check is dedicated to this process. But during that sound check, something interesting happens.

Essentially, many of the dials on that overwhelming sound board become more or less locked in. They're set to optimal levels, and now they don't have to be tweaked during the show, barring unforeseen circumstances. In the case of your health, "set it and forget it" can exist in the same way. When you can take advantage, the giant control board starts to feel less intimidating.

Here are the "set and forget" elements to your health protocol:
- How you eat
- How you move
- How you think
- How you sleep

You might read that and feel ripped off. And I get it: Starting a movement or exercise routine is difficult; eating well is sometimes harder. You might even be thinking that getting a handle on your thoughts and your sleep are the hardest parts of this. And that's an important distinction: I'm not saying that getting to where you need to be is easy in any of these categories.

Perhaps you have big lifestyle changes ahead, or ones that you're struggling with right now. But as a habit forms and eventually turns into a lifestyle, all of this gets easier. Eventually, your movement routine becomes almost automatic and your pantry is filled with nourishing foods. Don't rush the process—know that baby steps are okay. But when you arrive, you'll find it easier to maintain than it was initially to reach.

Embrace Seasons

If you think about the course of an entire year, you can probably pinpoint the reality that your lifestyle changes along with the seasons. If you have school-age kids, maybe you have a routine that incorporates packing lunches and arranging drop-offs. Depending on your routine, you might have more or less time to yourself at this time of year.

Summer rolls around and some parents are running kids to activities. Others are vacationing; some just cancel commitments and relax at home. A number of people work seasonally at this time. It should also be mentioned that millions deal with seasonal affective disorder in some regard. You might find yourself having a harder time finding motivation throughout your days in colder months, or that your mood shifts are more drastic then. Maybe you even enter a depressive state during that time.

It's outside the scope of this book to address the impact of seasonal shifts in their totality, but they are very real and each of us deals with them to some extent. Have some grace for yourself as you move throughout the seasons, and be aware of how your regular seasonal rhythms impact your perimenopause journey.

As routines change, embrace them to the best of your ability. Understand that your protocol should adapt along with you. There might be seasons when you need some extra support. Maybe you add a couple of supplements in the summer months that you don't take in the winter. Maybe quiet time doesn't come as easily in the fall and you need to be more intentional to schedule it in.

We're coming back to this concept of viewing your protocol as adaptable and anything but static. Instead of getting bogged down in the frustration of changing routines, embrace the seasons as they come!

Always Reevaluate the Products You Use

I don't stake my loyalty to any one supplement company. Over decades, I've found a few that I trust, but I encourage you to view each product as entirely different from the next. Instead of taking one vitamin D product and ditching it because you didn't see results, understand that the next vitamin D product you try might make a world of a difference. Why is this?

There is absolutely no standardization in the supplement industry. Since it's not regulated in the same way as prescription medicine, different manufacturers can have wildly different takes on how to formulate even basic products. I'm not asking you to become a supplement expert, but it is worth your time to have some basic knowledge.

Even if you select a quality product, just know that what works for me may not work for you! Don't bail out too early, but if you've gone three or four months and don't feel that you're seeing results or a particular product seems to disagree with you, switch to another product or brand of it! A different dosage, delivery method, key ingredient, cofactor, or potency could make all the difference.

You might try a couple of products (see the Resources section for a starting point) and have great success with one and no success at all with another. That's okay. This is not a prescription or an exact plan for success! I and other experts can give you ideas and point you in the right direction, but you should be okay with some experimentation here and there.

When You're at the End of Your Rope

No matter how successful your protocol, there may come days when you feel as if you're at the end of your rope. It could be that a new symptom flares up or an unexpected stressful situation arises, causing you to stumble three steps back. Or maybe you feel as if you've been grinding away without any success just yet.

That's okay. You're not alone.

When you feel that you've reached the end of the rope, the best way to keep moving forward is to fall back on the fundamentals. Instead of stressing about getting 20 minutes in the infrared sauna or starting up some new supplement, revisit the basics. Here's my recommended protocol for the worst days:

- Get outside
- Drink some water
- Move your body
- Sleep well

To get fancier, you know what I'm going to say. Check in on the state of your nervous system! You know it as well as me at this point—not one thing you're doing will make a positive impact if your body is in fight-or-flight survival mode. If you're stuck, please find someone you can lean on for support. Turn to someone for even a few minutes to serve as your substitute, so you can take a moment and reset. Hopefully a friend, spouse, child, or other family member can step up to the plate to support your health.

Respect that circadian rhythm we discussed earlier. Go outside into morning sunlight and cut off the blue screens earlier in the evening. I get that so-called doomscrolling is a coping mechanism, but you need to find better tools to help restore your mental sanity, if that's your only one.

But again, that feeling of being at the end of your rope? It's almost always a nervous system thing. If you're confident it isn't, that's a good time to explore these additional nutrients:

- Methylated B vitamins
- Magnesium
- CoQ10

If you do think that it could be a nervous system issue, know that you're not alone. Many people struggle to find balance when it feels as if their health is up in the air. Or worse yet, maybe you feel that your kids, your marriage, your job, your health, and everything else is up in the air. Have some grace for yourself within that.

You can't control it all, so focus on the variables you *can* control. Remember breathwork, quiet time, and the other tools that get you back to business.

Never Abandon Ship

Okay, so let's assume that things aren't going as planned in your healing journey. I encourage you to not abandon ship! Be mindful of the inhibiting factors that can cause an otherwise beneficial program to fail. You could be a tweak away from feeling like your best self. When a vessel on the ocean gets off course, the crew doesn't abandon ship, they make the necessary microadjustments to reorient themselves. You can and should do the same.

The hormone pathways we're working with are very sensitive. And if you're in perimenopause, you have at least a semblance of your menstrual cycle. Get this: Hormones can fluctuate by 25 percent within the course of a single day. And within the course of a cycle? Imagine how much they move. Some hormones (e.g., testosterone) should stay more consistent, but others (e.g., estrogen and progesterone) fluctuate greatly.

When it comes to the support you're providing, there are so many factors. Let's start with delivery method. Many of the hormone therapies I like to use are transdermal—could you try applying them to specific areas of the body, for better absorption? Timing could be an important element as well. Maybe you'd see better results applying certain therapies at the beginning or the end of the day. Some might go best with a meal or a snack.

Another tweak to consider is to make more moves to support liver health. We've already mentioned this idea, but let's get tactical. Previous chapters lay out concrete examples of ways to support your liver. Have you incorporated any? Hopefully, you have. If not, now's the time. Or, if you're incorporating a few of the gentler tactics, maybe it's time to consider twisting up the dial by adding a targeted supplement for additional support.

Trust me when I say the liver is often the linchpin. It's overwhelmed with numerous essential tasks to perform, and the work it does relating to hormones will often end up taking a backseat if the other tasks aren't being handled efficiently enough. There are ways to change the game for your liver health, and they're well worth exploring.

Understand that this is a dance, not a demolition. It goes back to the idea of the hormone symphony. If you've spent too much time working with the woodwinds and left the percussion section to itself, you might play again and find that the symphony still doesn't sound better. It doesn't mean you haven't done valuable work; it means that you need to go back to the table and evaluate all of the players, not just your pet projects.

Remember, this isn't a conversation strictly surrounding the sex hormones. Melatonin, insulin, cortisol, thyroid hormones, and vitamin D all sit at the table. Just one of these hormones being out of balance will disrupt the entire symphony. It's possible to see success. If you stick to a program, it's likely to see success—but that doesn't mean it's easy.

Sunsetting Perimenopause and Rising into Menopause

Wow, we've spent some time together fine-tuning your perimenopause journey. But at some point or another—spoiler alert—you will move into menopause. So, how do we transition successfully? The first goal is to understand what that transition entails. The factual difference is that the ovaries greatly reduce the production of estradiol. The medical definition of fully transitioning into menopause is the lack of a menstrual cycle for an entire year.

You'll probably know menopause is nearing as your cycles become extremely irregular—even more so than perimenopause acquainted you with. Maybe 50 days pass before the next cycle, then 60, then 90. You're not in menopause at this point, but you're nearing it and it's important to be mindful. Estradiol is pulling back as you go.

The good news is that the same tools apply during perimenopause and menopause. This book will still serve you well as you make that transition. However, there are a few key differences. For starters, this is when you might want to look at supporting your body's estrogen levels. If you recall, we took an unexpected hard left turn earlier in this book, when I brought up the fact that we don't supply added estrogens to the body during perimenopause in 9.9 out of 10 cases (even though others may advise it).

However, during *menopause*, estradiol or estriol could be valuable components in your health protocol. If you decide to pursue the option, I again encourage lab testing, to understand how your liver is clearing estrogens. If you've heard the chatter about estrogen dominance or hormone-sensitive cancers, you can rest easier knowing that the liver is doing its job and clearing out excess estrogen. If it isn't, that's when you find yourself with an elevated risk factor.

Blood Sugar Balance

Beyond estrogen, the goal is to continue to build metabolic flexibility. Blood sugar monitoring is a tool I like to introduce to women who are in menopause. Some women quantify this with continuous glucose monitors or first morning blood sugar monitoring. I'm not against those things and I think they can be valuable for a period of time, but I'd rather you learn to be intuitive with your body. Understand what balanced, low, and high blood sugar feel like to you.

Rising Cholesterol

Many women head into menopause only to find that their cholesterol is rising. Sometimes, this is the first time a woman has experienced this in their lifetime. It often happens without any dietary or lifestyle changes having been introduced. Why?

Earlier in this book, we introduced the hormone cascade. Think of it as a waterfall. At the top is a river: cholesterol. As it comes over the cliff, it transitions into a multitude of hormones, such as pregnenolone, progesterone, DHEA, testosterone, and estrogen. How weird is it that no one ever mentions the fact that hormones originate from cholesterol?

In menopause, you essentially have a beaver dam that's placed between cholesterol and pregnenolone. What happens then? The hormones start to dry up and cholesterol begins to pool. Explains a lot, right?

This is not a scare tactic, and this book is meant to ensure you that you're empowered at this point, but I do want you to understand the implications here. If you have a family history of cardiovascular disease, this pooling, left unchecked, creates risk factors for it to surface. By the way, it is my firm belief that cholesterol doesn't cause heart disease. However, if another factor, inflammation, is present—the stage is set for forming plaques, and other issues.

By the way, proper amounts of estradiol have been shown to increase HDL cholesterol, decrease LDL cholesterol, and decrease apolipoprotein B. Some encouragement with the reality that the moves you make can make a difference.

Bone Density

These hormonal changes also mean we need to be mindful of osteoporosis and osteopenia. Progesterone and estrogen are designed for something called osteoblastic activity. Basically, they're designed to build bone. On the other side of osteoblastic activity is osteoplastic activity—that's essentially the process of bones breaking down. The two together actually create a healthy cycle of bone production that's largely regulated by progesterone and estrogen.

When this process is out of balance, that's when osteopenia and osteoporosis are introduced. As lovingly as I can say this, you shouldn't need fancy medications for this—you just need hormone balance! I'm not advising you to disregard your doctor's good faith management of your individual circumstances, but I'm encouraging the vast majority of you that this can be managed inside your existing protocol without creating new worries and processes.

Brain Health

Dementia is one of the greatest fears of both men and women over the age of 50. I've had personal experiences with this nasty disease ravaging my own family, and I want to empower you to get ahead of it. Yes, unfortunately unmanaged menopause predisposes many women to dementia. In fact, 20 percent of women coming through menopause are currently being diagnosed with it.

Here's why that's happening. The frontal cortex—the executive function portion of your brain—is rich in estradiol receptors. By the way, the same goes for men. Instead of panicking, the best thing you can do is continue to support your body throughout all of menopause. Follow the same principles for healthy drainage that allow your body to clear toxins and things that are unneeded, offer hormonal support where you can, and, in general, stay in tune with your body!

Don't let fear or rose-colored glasses from influencers online drive you to taking 20 supplements right when you wake up. Trust me when I say women who have done this have come into my practice, and they're not feeling anything like they were promised. Stay the course, make the healthy decisions, and persevere.

It Takes a Team

As we come to the end of this book, I have to reflect on the fact that it takes a team to do almost anything substantial. I work alongside a dedicated team in my clinic who helped shape this book, and I'm grateful for the team our publisher has that refined it, got it into your hands, and brought it to life. But I use this example because it takes a team to navigate through perimenopause and, eventually, menopause.

Who's in your corner? First and foremost, if you're married—is your spouse supportive on the home front? For some, I cringe to ask because I know the feelings that must be stirred up if the answer to that question is uncertain or even a flat-out no. The decision to be supportive is not in your hands, and in many cases, our spouse doesn't step up to the plate in the way that we'd hoped. What then?

Put your health journey aside for a moment. Do you feel loved by your spouse apart from this? If so, you have a foundation in place that makes it possible to get that support you need. This is both an encouragement and a challenge for you and your partner—the women who come into my clinic with a supportive spouse have an exponentially better chance of getting well than do those who have a doubtful or discouraging spouse.

If you have tears in your eyes, wishing for a different circumstance, slow down for a moment. I'm not defending it, but many people misplace their love by using it to defend your current state. They cast doubt so you don't get your hopes up; they unknowingly sabotage you, so you stay in their comfort zone; . . . the list goes on. Sometimes, things like financial stress or different philosophies on wellness come into play. A lot of women choosing a natural, more comprehensive approach to wellness have to deal with partners who dismissively make the "Can't you just do X and be done with it?" commentary.

You're not alone, and you deserve to have the support of your spouse. Hopefully you're in a place where you feel comfortable having a sit-down conversation. Remind them how important they are to you and how far their support would go. Maybe they need you to hear out their concerns once, but ask them whether they can put their skepticism aside, to get in your corner.

Your spouse isn't the only member on your support team. And if you aren't married, this is the place to tune back in. Who else in life is in your corner? Do you have a trustworthy friend who never tires of being your support system? Parents or even adult children who have your back? Sometimes, even support groups can be a good option.

The point is to find people who can have your back and stand in your corner when you're ready to surrender. If you lack obvious choices for these roles, don't give up that easily. Find your community, so that you can press on. Make nervous system regulation easier by surrounding yourself with a group of people who remind you that you deserve this. When possible, connect with those around you who love and care about you. Don't become overly reliant on online personalities or influencers who broadcast messages without the ability to connect with you on a personal level.

The Body Is Designed to Work for You

I don't accept the prevailing views about the body. When it enters a diseased or stressed state, it is often the position of the medical community to believe that the body is flawed or broken. I, however, think differently. I believe with every fiber of my being that the body is designed to heal. What it needs is nothing in the way—no interference.

As you work on restoring your health, wellness, and life, remember that you're not at war with your body. You're clearing interference so that your body can resume its natural healing processes. You're not pursing a lab number on a chart, you're in the pursuit of *feeling* well. Would you rather feel like a new woman with some improvement in your lab reports or would you rather have perfect lab numbers and still feel as poorly as you do today?

The point is not to obsess over the quantification of everything. Trust yourself, trust how you feel, and trust your body.

Perimenopause itself isn't a problem, it's actually your opportunity. Despite the associations you have with it, perimenopause is nothing more than a chapter of your life. We get to be curious about it and build a toolset for it. You're not losing power, you're experiencing a turning point. In fact, you're stepping *into* power!

Your body isn't broken, but it might be asking for better care or better alignment.

Be Selfish Every Now and Then

Selfish is a word with some nasty connotations. When we think of selfish people, we think of the worst of us. But let me rattle the chain a little bit here—what if it's okay to be selfish? A woman came into my practice once, who told me that the closest translation for the world "selfish" in her language actually means "self-love." If you'd object to showing yourself love, there might be some work you have to do to remind yourself that you are worthy of it.

We even see this in the Bible. "Love your neighbor as yourself." The question I always have for women in shoes similar to yours is this: How are you doing at loving yourself? What does self-love look like for you? When you become capable of loving yourself, you become capable of being the full version of yourself. Loving yourself actually makes you more capable of being a better mom, friend, grandma, spouse, or girlfriend.

As a bonus, loving yourself helps ground your physical health. It puts you in a state where you can better receive everything we've put together in a protocol over these last six chapters.

Parting Words for You

My hope for you in completing this book is that you feel empowered. You have a toolbox for perimenopause and you're equipped for an eventual transition into menopause. Things will change, but you'll be ready for them. Improvements will come, and you'll be more aware of them. Challenges will arise, but you'll be ready for them.

This is a journey, and it's not always an easy one. There will be times when you want to give up. Don't let that happen. Persevere, tweak before you abandon ship, and stay the course when at all possible.

Sooner than you think, if you've taken each and every step seriously, you will have the opportunity to experience a remarkable transformation. Remember: Perimenopause isn't the time in every woman's life where the wheels fall off and things go crazy. Perimenopause and menopause are natural, gentle transitory periods that can be beautiful. Now that you've made it this far with me, I hope you'll employ the right tools to make that dream a reality for yourself.

Lean into the basics—get basic before you get fancy. You deserve to feel well, and I wholeheartedly believe that, in time, you will. If you find yourself enjoying life in a way you never thought you would again, please write to me. I'd love to celebrate that with you.

You've got this; now, let's go!

Resources & References

Resources
Find up-to-date, specific recommendations for supplements, labs, and other key resources at poweroverperimenopause.com.

References
1. "Perimenopause Fact Sheet: Jean Hailes for Women's Health," Jean Hailes, accessed April 25, 2025, www.jeanhailes.org.au/resources/perimenopause-fact-sheet.

2. Maunil K. Desai and Roberta Diaz Brinton, "Autoimmune Disease in Women: Endocrine Transition and Risk Across the Lifespan," *Frontiers in Endocrinology* 10, no. 265 (April 29, 2019), https://doi.org/10.3389/fendo.2019.00265.

3. "Childhood Trauma & ACES," Cleveland Clinic, July 16, 2025, accessed September 14, 2025, my.clevelandclinic.org/health/symptoms/24875-adverse-childhood-experiences-ace.

4. Ming Tai-Seale et al., "Time Allocation In Primary Care Office Visits," *Health Services Research* 42, no. 5 (2007): 1871–94, https://doi.org/10.1111/j.1475-6773.2006.00689.x.

5. "Sympathetic Nervous System (SNS)," Cleveland Clinic, June 6, 2022, accessed May 8, 2025, my.clevelandclinic.org/health/body/23262-sympathetic-nervous-system-sns-fight-or-flight.

6. Gilian Crowther, "The Cell Danger Response: A New Paradigm for Understanding Chronic Disease?" *IHCAN Mitochondrial Medicine* (2018): 30–34, accessed 5 May 5, 2025, https://aonm.org/wp-content/uploads/2021/07/Cell-Danger-Response-IHCAN.pdf.

7. Matthew Solan, "Tired? 4 Simple Ways to Boost Energy," *Harvard Health Blog*, Harvard Health Publishing, September 7, 2018, accessed April 30, 2025, www.health.harvard.edu/blog/tired-4-simple-ways-to-boost-energy-2018090714678.

8. Kimberly Y. Z. Forrest and Wendy L. Stuhldreher. "Prevalence and Correlates of Vitamin D Deficiency in US Adults," *Nutrition Research* (New York). 31, no. 1 (2011): 48–54, https://doi.org/10.1016/j.nutres.2010.12.001.

9. "Menopausal Hormone Therapy and Cancer Risk," American Cancer Society, February 13, 2015, accessed September 15, 2025, www.cancer.org/cancer/risk-prevention/medical-treatments/menopausal-hormone-replacement-therapy-and-cancer-risk.html.

Acknowledgments

This book, *Power Over Perimenopause*, is the fruit of years of passion, purpose, and the people who've stood beside me through it all. I would be nowhere without the support, sacrifice, and belief of those closest to me.

Rachel, my wife of 24 years—you are the fierce love behind every risk I've taken and every dream I've dared to chase. No one has ever believed in me like you do. You've seen the gifts God placed inside me even when I doubted them. You've carried our home, our family, and so much more so I could pour myself into this mission. Your strength is unmatched. Thank you for being the anchor and the fire. I love you deeply.

To my children—Adrienne, Jayden, Breck, Lynnlee, and Navia—you are the light of my eye. Your unconditional love, your grace, your excitement, your presence . . . it's been fuel for my soul in the hardest and holiest moments. I love being "front door famous" to you more than any accolade I'll ever receive. Watching you grow up into who God made you to be fills me with pride. My prayer is that you'll one day stand on the shoulders of your mom and me and run even farther than we ever could. May your lives overflow with love, joy, peace, patience, kindness, gentleness, faithfulness, and self-control.

To my Creator—everything starts and ends with You. Years ago, You spoke to me: "You are a Revealer of People's Potential." I've held that truth tightly ever since. John 10:10 reminds me that You came to give life—and not just any life, but life to the full. That's what this book is about. That's what my life's work is about. Thank You for Your guidance, Your grace, and the calling You've given me.

To my team at Dr. Greg–Functional Medicine—Lauren, Loredana, Courtney, Maribeth, CC, Heidi, Ben, Eric, and Adrienne—this clinic exists because of your commitment to serving well. Your dedication to our patients is unmatched. I've watched you show up day in and day out with compassion, grit, and excellence. The lives we've touched, the healing we've helped usher in—it's all because you decided to be part of something bigger than yourselves. I'm honored to serve alongside you.

Eric Johnson—The time you spent with me dreaming of writing a book, sitting with me crafting the message, interviewing me for podcasts will never be forgotten. You are a true friend, and I am grateful for our brotherhood. You're also the guy who nudged me to post a TikTok over five years ago, which sparked a movement. Your heart to serve others, your clarity in communication, and your behind-the-scenes sacrifice have made this book possible. You've helped take scattered thoughts from conversations and shape them into a message that now lives on paper. Thank you for walking with me.

To everyone at Page Street Publishing—I can say with confidence that this book would not exist without the unique expertise each and every member of the team brought to the process. You are the best of the best at what you do. To my editor, Marissa Giambelluca, thank you for taking a chance on a first-time author and for your patience guiding the process, quelling concerns, and refining the message. Thank you for forwarding the concept that ultimately led to this book.

To everyone who has read, listened, shared, and supported—this is for you. I wrote this book because I believe with everything in me that women deserve to feel empowered, seen, and equipped.

About the Author

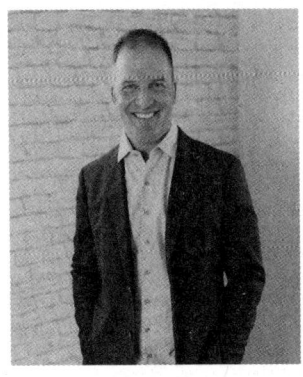

Dr. Greg Mongeon helped introduce the world to a better path toward health and healing. Tens of millions have tuned in to join him on one of his famous "walk and talks" on social media, and thousands have stepped into his clinic to benefit from a novel approach that considers the root cause. The people-centric approach he developed set a new standard for what it means to receive care.

Dr. Greg's adamant belief is that the body is designed to heal—it just needs to be free from interference. His philosophy drives his clinical practice: Dr. Greg–Functional Medicine. At the clinic, he and his team spearhead an unprecedented model of unlimited access where patients aren't billed on a per-appointment basis but instead encouraged to reach out as often as needed.

At home, Dr. Greg is a dedicated husband and father to five kids. He is relentlessly in pursuit of optimal health—spiritually, emotionally, mentally, and physically.

Index

A
abdominal self-massage, 45
absorptivity, 126
acetyl-L-carnitine (ALC), 37, 117
acne, cystic, 167
adaptogens, 129
adrenal glands, 165
adrenal lab tests, 103
advanced therapies, 168
adverse childhood experiences (ACEs), 165, 185
aging, 13
alpha lipoic acid (ALA), 37, 46, 117
American Cancer Society, 120
androgen, 86
anemia, low-level, 157
anemia lab test, 104
antioxidants, 36–37, 118
antiperspirants, 47, 117
anxiety, 63, 158
apolipoprotein B, 178
aromatase, 86
ATP, 31–32, 34
autoimmune disease, 16, 185

B
B vitamins, methylated, 174
basophils, 167
bioidentical hormone therapy (BHRT), 73–75, 79, 81, 120
birth control, 72, 81
bisphenol A (BPA), 115
bitters, 153
blood sugar, 159, 164, 177
blue light exposure, 40, 167
bone density, 179
bowel function, 43–45
bowel movements, 77, 118
box breathing, 28, 48, 133, 152
brain fog, 27
brain health, 179–80
breaks, 169
breast fullness, 159
breast tenderness, 159
breath holding, 152
breathwork, 28–29, 41, 133, 152
Brinton, Roberta Diaz, 16

C
C-reactive protein, high-sensitivity (HS-CRP), 103
caffeine, 133–34
castor oil packs, 44, 134, 155
CBC lab tests, 167
cell danger response (CDR), 31, 185
cellular energy, 31–32, 153
cholesterol, 51, 86–87, 178
chronic illness, 146–47, 185
circadian rhythms, 167–68, 174
Cleveland Clinic, 18
cognitive patterns, 170
    mindset, 149, 166–67
communication
    self-talk, 25, 149, 169
    with your spouse or partner, 148–51, 181
comprehensive metabolic profile (CMP), 105, 115
computer screens, 40, 167
constipation, 63, 118
CoQ10, 174
cortisol, 51, 54–55, 129, 158, 176
culture, 12–13

D
daily walks, 117–18
date nights, 155
dehydroepiandrosterone (DHEA), 51, 76, 86, 91, 106, 109, 128, 166–67, 178
dementia, 179–80
deodorants, 47
depression, 27
Desai, Maunil K., 16
detoxification, 45, 117–18, 134, 144, 146, 159, 167–68
DHEA (dehydroepiandrosterone), 51, 76, 86, 91, 106, 109, 166–67, 178
DHEA replenishment, 128
dietary modifications, 33–35
    healthy eating, 134
    standard American diet (S.A.D.), 57
digestive issues, 63, 153
Dirty Dozen, 68–69
dorsal vagal shutdown, 27–28
drainage & energy protocol, 115–19, 136
drainage lab test, 104–5
drainage promotion, 29, 41–48, 110, 144, 164
    signs of poor drainage, 43
    support tactics, 44–48, 118, 134
    troubleshooting, 48
drainage supplements, 118
dry brushing, 46, 134, 155

E
endocrine-disrupting chemicals (EDCs), 64–69, 159
endocrine disruptors. see endocrine-disrupting chemicals (EDCs)
energy, 29, 32–41
    cellular, 31–32, 153
    drainage & energy protocol, 115–19, 136
    tools for boosting, 153, 185
Environmental Working Group (EWG), 68–69
enzymes, digestive, 153
estradiol (E2), 74, 86, 176–78
estriol, 177
estrogen, 52–53, 63, 86–89, 114, 178–79
    xenoestrogens, 159
estrogen deficiency, 64, 89, 157, 159
estrogen dominance, 50, 159
estrogen excess, 89
exercise, 37–38
exhalation, forced, 152

F
Factor V Leiden, 80
fasting insulin test, 102

fatigue, 27, 157
fatty acids, 35, 117
fight-or-flight responses, 26–27, 111, 119
fluid intake, 33, 45, 118, 173
food(s)
   Dirty Dozen, 68–69
   fatty acid sources, 35
   healthy eating, 134, 170
   protein sources, 34
   before sleeping, 39–40
   tracking, 154
forced exhalation, 152
forever chemicals, 64–67
fragrance, 68
friends, 23–24, 180–82
functional medicine, 19–22

G

gallbladder, 70–71
glucose, 57
glucose monitors, 159, 177
glutathione, 118, 154
glymphatic system, 40, 46–47
gratitude journal, 40
Graves' disease, 58
gut health, 164
   key tactics for, 44–45, 144
   support tools, 153
gut inflammation, 158
gym routines, 38

H

habits, 170
Harvard Health Blog, 34
Hashimoto's thyroiditis, 58
Hawaii, 130
HDL cholesterol, 178
Health Services Research, 21
health trends, 168
healthy eating, 134
hemoglobin, 157
herbal supplements, 45
herbicides, 68–69
high-sensitivity C-reactive protein (HS-CRP), 103
histamine intolerance, 158
hormonal resilience, 163–65
hormone balance, 60–61, 176
   imbalance, 50, 70–71, 141
   optimizing, 75, 79–80, 92, 100, 106

perimenopause fluctuations, 6, 17, 22, 174
perimenopause ripple effect, 62–64
postpartum fluctuations, 15
protocol for, 120–22
puberty fluctuations, 14–15
symptoms due to, 96–99
hormone cascade, 50–51, 86–87, 178
hormone deficiency, 141, 145–46
hormone replacement therapy (HRT), 21, 72–74
hormone resistance, 106–7
hormone supplements, 76
hormone therapy, 122–27, 145
   additional, 127–30, 136–37
   delivery methods, 126, 175
   interactions, 144
   resources for, 185
Hormone Zoomer panel, 114–15
hormones, 49–82
   bioidentical, 73–75, 79, 81, 120
   lab tests for, 100–101, 105, 108, 114
   sex, 100–101, 129
   synthetic, 72–73
   thyroid, 76–77, 81, 92, 128, 176
hot flashes, 144, 159
household products
   endocrine-disrupting chemicals (EDCs), 64–69, 159
   top products to swap out, 67–69
hydration, 33, 45, 118, 173
hydrochloric acid, 153
hyperthyroidism, 58
hypothalamic-pituitary-adrenal axis, 157
hypothyroidism, 58, 158

I

Ideal Day exercise, 84–85
imitators, 156–59
in vitro fertilization (IVF), 71
inflammation, 158, 178
inflammatory lab test, 103
infrared saunas, 134, 155

insomnia, 39
Instagram, 13, 23–24
insulin, 57–58, 66, 176
   fasting, 102
   symptoms caused by, 94
insulin resistance, 57–58, 94, 106, 158
irritability, 158

J

journaling, 40–41, 154

K

kidneys, 45–46

L

lab tests, 13, 77–79, 99–106, 141
   adrenal, 103
   anemia, 104
   CBC, 167
   comprehensive, 99, 105, 109, 115
   correlating with symptoms, 109, 114–15
   drainage, 104–5
   hormone, 100–101, 105, 108, 115
   Hormone Zoomer, 114–15
   in-range, 77
   inflammatory, 103
   during menopause, 177
   metabolic, 102, 115
   methylation, 104
   optimal numbers, 108–9
   ordering, 110
   resources for, 185
   vs. symptoms, 99, 109
   thyroid, 101–2
   vitamin D, 103
   when to have, 107–8
LDL cholesterol, 178
lies, 12–13
life accumulation, 14, 17–18
lifestyle changes, 20–21, 29, 81–82, 170
   key practices, 133–35
   tools for, 155
liver support, 45–46, 70–71, 116, 118, 141, 144, 159, 175
   tools for, 154
low libido, 17
luteal phase, 107–8

lymphatic drainage, 134
lymphatic massage, 46, 134
lymphatic system, 46–47

M

magnesium, 144, 174
manageable movement, 38
managed care, 145–46
massage
    abdominal self-massage, 45
    lymphatic, 46, 134
melatonin, 55–56, 81, 108, 176
    low, 95
    symptoms caused by, 94–95
melatonin replenishment, 129
men, 149–51
menopause, 184
    definition of, 23, 176
    vs. perimenopause, 22–23
    transition into, 176–80
menstrual cycle, 144
    responsiveness to, 142
    tracking, 154
metabolic lab tests, 102, 105, 115
metabolic resilience, 163–65
methylation lab test, 104
microadjustments, 139
micronutrients, 144, 166
milk thistle, 118
mindset, 149, 166–67
misconceptions, 12–13
misdiagnoses, 156–59
mitochondria, 31
mitochondrial support supplements, 36–37, 117–18, 153
mood swings, 17, 154
morning routines, 133, 168
mouth taping, 41
movement routines, 38, 46, 170, 173
MTHFR, 146

N

n-acetyl cysteine (NAC), 37, 46, 117
natural family planning, 52
natural supplements, 76–77
nature activity, 173
Naviaux, Robert, 31
nebulizers, 48

nervous system
    fight-or-flight responses, 26–27, 111, 119
    frozen, 27–28
nervous system regulation, 119, 136, 164, 166, 181–82
    with breathwork, 28–29
    tools for, 152
night sweats, 159
nutraceuticals, 126
nutrients, 174
    micronutrients, 144, 166
nutrition, 45, 153

O

osteoblastic activity, 179
osteopenia, 179
osteoporosis, 179
outdoor activity, 173
over-the-counter supplements, 154

P

parasites, 167
parasympathetic nervous system, 28
PCOS (polycystic ovary syndrome), 58
Peatross, Jess, 6–7
perimenopause, 6–8, 17, 163, 182, 184
    definition of, 22–23
    framework for, 110–11
    hormone ripple effect in, 62–64
    keys for long-term success, 162–84
    vs. menopause, 22–23
    resources for, 185
    transition into menopause from, 176–80
    Ultimate Perimenopause Symptoms Checklist, 87–95, 135, 142, 152, 156
personal care, 141–42
pesticides, 68–69
PFAs, 65
physical activity, 45–46, 155, 170
    daily walks, 117–18
    manageable movement, 38
    for the worst days, 173
pineal gland, 40

plan B, 145–46
polycystic ovary syndrome (PCOS), 58
poop, 43–44, 154
prayer, 40–41
pregnenolone, 51, 76, 86, 178
progesterone, 51, 53, 75, 77, 86–87, 178–79
progesterone deficiency, 63, 90, 124–25, 158
progesterone excess, 91
progesterone products, 127
progesterone replenishment, 128, 142
protein, 34–35, 117–18, 134
puberty, 14–15

R

resources, 185
respiratory system, 47–48
resveratrol, 37, 117

S

saunas, infrared, 134, 155
seasonal affective disorder, 171
seasonal shifts, 171–72
self-care, 132, 141–42, 183
self-love, 183
self-talk, 25, 149, 169
selfishness, 183
senna leaf, 45
sex hormone lab tests, 100–101
sex hormones, 129
silymarin, 118
sleep hygiene, 39–41, 46–47, 117–18, 164, 170
    recommendations for, 39–40
    for the worst days, 173
Sloan, Matthew, 34
social media, 23–24, 133
soy, 73
standard American diet (S.A.D.), 57
State of the Union exercise, 24–26, 78–79, 85–86, 107, 114, 137, 152, 154
stress
    evaluation of, 130–32, 135–36, 143
    life accumulation, 17–18

stress management, 130–32, 135–36, 143, 152
stress reduction, 81–82, 119, 143
supplements, 21, 33–37, 180
    for bowel function, 44–45
    drainage, 118
    herbal, 45
    hormone, 76
    for kidney and liver support, 46
    for mitochondrial support, 36–37, 117–18, 153
    natural, 76–77
    over-the-counter, 154
    re-evaluation of, 172–73
    resources for, 185
    vitamin D, 57, 81
support systems, 180–82
sweat glands, 47–48
sympathetic nervous system, 26, 185
symptoms
    causes of, 16–17
    correlating with lab tests, 114–15
    of estrogen deficiency, 89
    of estrogen excess, 89
    hormones, 96–99
    imitators, 156–59
    of insulin resistance, 94
    vs. lab tests, 99, 109
    of low melatonin, 95
    of low vitamin D, 95
    misdiagnoses, 156–59
    of overactive thyroid, 93
    progesterone deficiency, 142
    of progesterone deficiency, 90
    of progesterone excess, 91
    signals, 97–99
    of testosterone deficiency, 91–92
    of testosterone excess, 92
    Ultimate Perimenopause Symptoms Checklist, 87–95, 135, 142, 152, 156
    of underactive thyroid, 93
synthetic hormones, 72–73

T

T3, 59, 77, 101–2
T4, 59, 77, 101–2
tauroursodeoxycholic acid (TUDCA), 46, 116
teamwork, 180–82
testosterone, 53–54, 60, 75–77, 86–87, 106, 178
testosterone deficiency, 91–92, 157, 166–67
testosterone excess, 92
testosterone replenishment, 128
thinking patterns, 170
thyroid, 51, 93
thyroid hormones, 58–59, 76–77, 81, 92, 128, 176
thyroid lab tests, 101–2
thyroid stimulating hormone (TSH), 58–59
thyroid symptoms, 92–93
TikTok, 13, 23–24
time management, 131–35, 155, 185
toxins, 45, 117–18
trauma, 146, 185
troubleshooting, 146–56

U

Ultimate Perimenopause Symptoms Checklist, 87–95, 135, 142, 152, 156
urinary tract infections (UTIs), 17

V

vitamin A deficiency, 51, 166
vitamin B12, 161
vitamin B12 deficiency, 157
vitamin D, 56–57, 176
vitamin D deficiency, 56–57, 64, 95, 130, 185
vitamin D lab test, 103
vitamin D replenishment, 129–30
vitamin D supplements, 57, 81
Vitamin D3, 130
vitamin K2, 57, 130

W

walks, daily, 117–18
water intake, 116
weight gain, 158
weight loss, 13
wellness protocols
    for drainage & energy, 115–19, 136
    end goal, 163–65
    for hormone balance, 120–22
    key for long-term success, 162–84
    key practices, 133–35
    overhauling, 151–56
    for seasonal changes, 171–72
    "set and forget" elements, 170
    seven steps, 135–37
    tools for, 151–56
    troubleshooting, 146–51, 165–69
    for the worst days, 173
Western medicine, 19–20, 61, 87, 182
white blood cells (WBCs), 167
wild yams, 73, 126
WorldLink Medical Academy, 79, 121

X

xenoestrogens, 159

Y

Yuka, 69